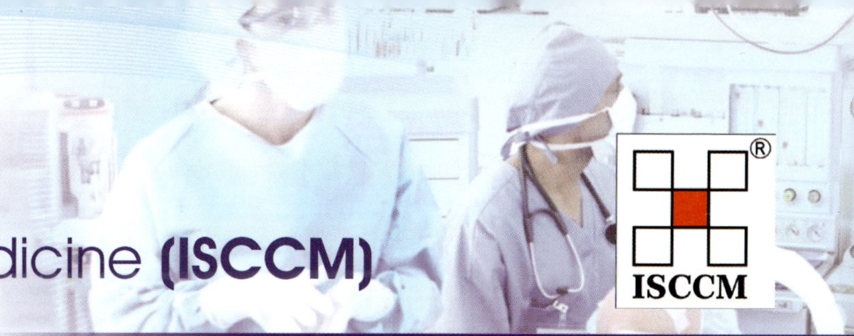

Indian Society of
Critical Care Medicine (ISCCM)

21 Common Diagnoses in ICU

A Case Based Approach

Indian Society of Critical Care Medicine (ISCCM)

ISCCM

21 Common Diagnoses in ICU

A Case Based Approach

Editors

Jorge Hidalgo MD MACP MCCM FCCP
Professor of Critical Care
Head of the General ICU and COVID-19 Unit
Belize Healthcare Partners Limited
President-Elect, World Federation of Intensive and Critical Care

Rajesh Chandra Mishra
MBBS MD (Medicine) FNBCCM
EDICM FCCM FICCM FCCP FICP
Consultant Intensivist and Internist,
Shaibya Comprehensive Care Clinic, Ahmedabad
Tele-ICU Expert
Medical Congress Advisor

Ahsina Jahan Lopa MBBS FICM
Incharge, Department of ICU and Emergency
Shahabuddin Medical College Hospital
Dhaka, Bangladesh

CBSPD

CBS Publishers & Distributors Pvt Ltd

New Delhi • Bengaluru • Chennai • Kochi • Kolkata • Lucknow • Mumbai
Gujarat • Hyderabad • Jharkhand • Nagpur • Patna • Pune • Uttarakhand

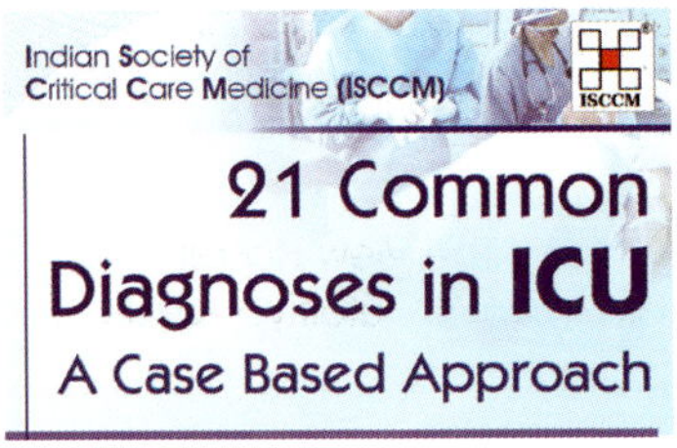

ISBN: 978-93-5466-699-5

First Edition: 2026

Published by Satish Kumar Jain and produced by Varun Jain for
CBS Publishers & Distributors Pvt Ltd
4819/XI Prahlad Street, 24 Ansari Road, Daryaganj, New Delhi 110 002, India
Ph: 011-23289259, 23266838 Website: www.cbspd.com
e-mail: delhi@cbspd.com

Corporate Office: 204 FIE, Industrial Area, Patparganj, Delhi 110 092, India
Ph: 011-49344934 Fax: 011-49344935 e-mail: publishing@cbspd.com; publicity@cbspd.com

Branches

- **Bengaluru:** Seema House 2975, 17th Cross, KR Road, Banasankari 2nd Stage, Bengaluru 560 070, Karnataka, India
  Ph: +91-80-26771678/79 Fax: +91-80-26771680 e-mail: bangalore@cbspd.com
- **Chennai:** 18/8B, Subbarayan Street, Shenoy Nagar, Chennai 600 030, Tamil Nadu, India
  Ph: +91-44-42032115, 45022115 e-mail: chennai@cbspd.com
- **Kochi:** 42/1325, 1326, Power House Road, Opposite KSEB, Kochi 682018, Kerala, India
  Ph: +91-484-4059061–65 Fax: +91-484-4059065 e-mail: kochi@cbspd.com
- **Kolkata:** 147, Hind Ceramics Compound, 1st Floor, Nilgunj Road, Belghoria, Kolkata 700056, West Bengal, India
  Ph: +91-33-25633055/56 e-mail: kolkata@cbspd.com
- **Lucknow:** Basement, Khushnuma Complex, 7 Meerabai Marg (behind Jawahar Bhawan), Lucknow 226001, UP, India
  Ph: +91-522-4000032 e-mail: tiwari.lucknow@cbspd.com
- **Mumbai:** PWD Shed, Gala No. 25/26, Ramchandra Bhatt Marg, Next JJ Hospital Gate No. 2, Opp. Union Bank of India, Noorbaug, Mumbai 400009, Maharashtra, India
  Ph: +91-22-66661880/89 e-mail: mumbai@cbspd.com

Representatives

- **Gujarat** • **Hyderabad** • **Jharkhand** • **Nagpur** • **Patna** • **Pune** • **Uttarakhand**

For trade terms please contact customercare@cbspd.com
For general enquiries please contact info@cbspd.com

Printed at: Goyal Offset Works Pvt. Ltd., Kundli, Haryana, India

Contributors

Ahsan Ahmed MBBS DA DNB IFCCM EDIC
Assistant Professor
Anesthesiology and Chief of Critical Care and Emergency Services, KPC Medical College and Hospital, Kolkata

Ahsina Jahan Lopa MBBS FICM
Incharge, Department of ICU and Emergency
Shahabuddin Medical College Hospital
Dhaka, Bangladesh

Allyson Hidalgo
Biochemistry, Arizona State University
Phoenix AZ, USA

Ángel Augusto Pérez Calatayud
Jefe de división de Medicina Crítica Hospital General de México
Delegación Cuauhtémoc

Ansuka Mudalige
MBBS MD (Anaesthesiology) FRCA FFICM EDIC
Consultant Intensivist, Colombo North Teaching Hospital, Sri Lanka

Ashish K Khanna MD MS FCCP FCCM FASA
Associate Professor, Vice-Chair of Research
Director Perioperative Outcomes and Informatics Collaborative at Wake Forest School of Medicine and Atrium Health Wake Forest Baptist Medical Center
Winston Salem, NC 27106

Barnabe Carrillo
Neuro Interventional Radiologist Fellow
Far Eastern Memorial Hospital, New Taipei, Taiwán

Carlos Sanchez
Jefe de la Unidad de Cuidados Intensivos del Hospital General IESS Quevedo
Ecuador

Cassidy Vigil
PA-C, MMS
APP VAD/Transplant Coordinator in Advanced Heart Failure at Atrium Health Wake Forest Baptist Medical Center
Winston Salem, NC 27106

Dipanjan Chatterjee MD FNB
Head
Cardiopulmonary Critical Care
Director, ECMO and Transplant Program
Medica Superspeciality Hospital, Kolkata, India

Divya Shetty

Erika P. Plata-Menchaca
Critical Care Department. The View Hospital-in Affiliation with Cedars Sinai, Al Qutaifiya Area, Doha, Qatar

Gandra D'Almeida A MD EMDM FCCM FACS
OF-3 Moreno R., Phd, Portugal

Gentle Sunder Shrestha
Associate Professor
Department of Critical Care Medicine
Department of Critical Care Medicine, Tribhuvan University Teaching Hospital, Maharajgunj, Kathmandu, Nepal

Gloria Rodríguez-Vega
MD FACP FCCP FNCS MCCM
Chief, Department of Critical Care
Director, Neurosurgical ICU
HIMA-San Pablo-Caguas
Puerto Rico

Huda Al Khalili
Consultant Critical Care
Royal Hospital, Muscat, Oman

Javier Perez-Fernandez
Medical Director, Critical Care Services, Baptist Hospital of Miami
Director Critical Care Fellowship Training Program
Larkin Palm-Springs Hospital
Secretary General World Federation Intensive and Critical Care (WFICC)
Paola Perez
University of Virginia, School of Medicine

Jorge Hidalgo
MD MACP MCCM FCCP
Professor of Critical Care
Head of the General ICU and COVID-19 Unit at Belize Healthcare Partners Limited
President-Elect, World Federation of Intensive and Critical Care

Juhi Chandwani
Consultant Critical Care
Royal Hospital
Muscat, Oman

Kathryn Essak

Lilanthi Subasinghe
MD (Medicine) SRI LANKA,3. MRCP (UK), EDIC
University Hospital–General Sir John Kotelawala Defence University, Sri Lanka

Lillie Pitts MD
Medical Center Blvd
Winston-Salem, NC 27103

Marcio Borges Sa
Multidisicplinary Sepsis Unit, Intensive Care Unit
Carretera de Manacor, km 4
Son Llatzer University Hospital,
Palma de Mallorca, Spain

Maria Ortega Alaminos
Multidisicplinary Sepsis Unit, Son Llatzer University Hospital, Palma de Mallorca, Spain
Intensive Care Unit, Son Llatzer University Hospital, Palma de Mallorca, Spain
Multidisciplinary Sepsis Group, Health Research Institute of the Balearic Islands

Monika Gulati

Moreno R

Mudalige AD

Namalie KD
MBBS Diploma (Med Micro) MD (Med Micro)
Consultant Microbiologist, Colombo North Teaching Hospital, Sri Lanka

Nitin Arora

Paola Perez

Pedro Arriaga

Quirino Piacevoli MD PhD
Professor and Head, Department of Anesthesia and Intensive Care, ACO San Filippo Neri
Visiting Professor University "Campus Bio Medico"
Rome–Italy

Rajesh Chandra Mishra
MBBS MD (Medicine) FNBCCM
EDICM FCCM FICCM FCCP FICP
Consultant Intensivist and Internist,
Shaibya Comprehensive Care Clinic, Ahmedabad
Tele-ICU Expert
Medical Congress Advisor

Ricard Ferrer
Intensive Care Department, Hospital Universitari Vall d´Hebron, Vall d´Hebron
Shock, Organ Dysfunction and Resuscitation Group of Research, Vall d´Hebron Institute of Research
Vall d´Hebron Hospital Campus

Sachit Sharma

Sandeep Kantor MD FCCM FICCM
Consultant Critical Care
Royal Hospital, Muscat, Oman

Sharmili Sinha MD DNB EDIC FICCM
Senior Consultant, Critical Care
Apollo Hospitals, Bhubaneswar, India

Shashi Bhaskara Krishnamurthy
MBBS FCARCSI (Ireland) FCICM (Australia and NZ) MHA (Australia)
Director of Clinical Education and Intensivist
Cloudphysician Healthcare Private Limited
Bengaluru

Tarun Kapoor MD
Critical Care Fellow
Alpharetta GA 30005

Veronica Lisseth Hernandez González
Multidisicplinary Sepsis Unit, Son Llatzer University Hospital, Palma de Mallorca, Spain
Intensive Care Unit, Son Llatzer University Hospital
Palma de Mallorca, Spain

Vivek Gupta DA DNB FIACTA FICCM
Consultant Cardiac Anaesthesia and Intensive Care
Hero DMC Heart Institute Ludhiana
Punjab, India

Preface

We are delighted to introduce *21 Common Diagnoses in ICU: A Case Based Approach*, which provides the physician with a guide to both the approach to the patient and the treatment in a case-based approach. The way we address our patient care, teaching, and critical care investigation are energized fundamentally by our clinical practice. In turn, our practice is informed, animated, and balanced by the information and environment arising around learning and research. Clinical excellence is founded on careful history-taking and a complete physical examination, complemented by proper laboratory testing. These data raise questions concerning the patient's disease mechanisms, upon which a comprehensive, prioritized differential diagnosis is formulated and a treatment plan initiated. The reality and complexity of the clinical cases in the ICU drive our search for a better understanding of pathophysiology of critical care and new and effective therapies. We hope this textbook reflects the interconnection and mutually supporting threads of critical care practice, teaching, and research.

In this book, we intend to present a precise definition of diseases as this allows accurate diagnosis, which is essential to enable appropriate therapeutic interventions and maximize outcomes. Some medical conditions have fairly clear-cut pathophysiology, which is simple to define and diagnose and can be made in the presence of comparatively specific clinical symptoms and supported by images and laboratory testing. However, in the ICU setting, we face a very complex clinical scenario every day. Our understanding of the various microorganisms, the different age groups, medical backgrounds, predisposing factors, and genetic traits, among others, results in varying degrees of immune response.

We are working with an outstanding group of physicians and researchers worldwide. We have led an effort to present 21 *common diagnoses in ICU*. We want to thank all the authors for their excellent contributions. We hope all the readers will have a good time of reading this book.

Jorge Hidalgo
Rajesh Chandra Mishra
Ahsina Jahan Lopa

Contents

CHAPTER

1

Severe COVID-19 Infection

Rajesh Chandra Mishra, Sharmili Sinha, Vivek Gupta

CASE PRESENTATION

A 37-year-old male patient without any previous medical history was admitted to emergency department with difficulty in breathing for the last few hours; he also reported high grade fever, sore throat and generalized weakness for last 3–4 days. On evaluation, he was febrile (101°F), tachypnoic, using his accessory muscle for breathing and his oxygen saturation was 84%. He was a chronic smoker and using 2 packs/day. He was immediately started with oxygen using nonrebreathing mask. A rapid antigen testing was positive for Covid-19 infection. Blood investigations were sent immediately along with C-reactive protein (CRP), D-dimer and a chest X-ray was done. His oxygen saturation did not improve and he remained tachypnic. He was supported with noninvasive ventilation with increasing oxygen and ventilatory support, however, he remained hypoxemic and his work of breathing remained high with subcostal retraction. His arterial blood gases showed mixed respiratory failure (pH 7.12, $PaCO_2$ 59, PaO_2 54). He was started with Remdesivir and steroids. He was electively intubated and mechanically ventilated. In the next few hours his oxygenation did not improve in spite of increasing positive end expiratory pressure (PEEP) and keeping fraction of inspired oxygen FiO_2 1.0. He required small dose norepinephrine infusion (0.05 µg/kg/min) to maintain his blood pressure after adequate fluid administration. His blood gases further worsened with PaO_2: FiO_2 48, hypercapnea despite ventilator rate of 28, with plateau pressure 42. In the last 2 hours his urine output started falling and his lactate levels were 4.1 mmol/L.

Q. How Adequate Oxygenation can be Maintained and what other Strategies should be followed to Optimize this Patient?

The clinical spectrum of patients with Covid-19 infection ranges from no symptoms to critical illness. However, clinical condition of patient may overlap and may change over time. The patients with severe illness present with SpO_2 <94% on room air, arterial partial pressure of oxygen to fraction of inspired oxygen (PaO_2/FiO_2) <300 mm Hg, a respiratory rate >30 breaths/min, or lung infiltrates >50%. However, these patients may further worsen and nearly 5% of all covid infected patients become critical and require ICU admission.[1] These patients may develop respiratory failure, distributive shock, and/or involvement of other organs leading to multiple organ dysfunction. Patients aged ≥65 years or who are having bronchial asthma or chronic respiratory disease, malignancy, cardiovascular disease, chronic renal or hepatic disease, diabetes, advanced or untreated HIV infection, obesity, pregnancy, cigarette smoking or post-transplant are at higher risk for progressing to severe or critical disease.[2] Almost two-thirds of the patients admitted in ICU develop acute hypoxemic respiratory failure. All the patients who require oxygen therapy above 6–8 L/min to achieve oxygen saturation around 90–92%, or develop respiratory failure, shock, acute organ dysfunction and at risk of clinical deterioration should be admitted in ICU. Patients with hyperpyrexia, above 65 years of age, increased acute-phase reactants such as C–reactive protein and serum ferritin, lymphocytopenia, altered hepatic enzymes, increased D-dimer or acute kidney injury are prone for developing ARDS.[3]

ARDS is primarily non-cardiogenic inflammatory pulmonary edema, with reduced area of normal ventilation in lungs with reduced lung compliance and shunt effect. Berlin definition defines ARDS on the basis of degree of hypoxemia: Mild (200 mmHg < PaO_2/FIO_2 ≤300 mmHg), moderate (100 mmHg <PaO_2/FIO_2 ≤200 mmHg), and severe (PaO_2/FIO_2 ≤100 mmHg) along with radiographic severity, lung compliance (≤40 mL/cm H_2O), requirement of PEEP (positive end-expiratory pressure) ≥10 cm H_2O, and corrected expired volume per minute (≥10 L/min).[4] The COVID-19-induced ARDS patients have intense endothelial dysfunction and thromboinflammatory response. This may lead to abolition of hypoxic pulmonary vasoconstriction (HPV), severe pulmonary vasoconstriction and formation of micro or macrothrombus. These all contribute to increasing dead space, V/Q (ventilation/perfusion) mismatch leading to inadequate gas exchange and vasodilation.[5]

In patients admitted in ICU with severe gas exchange abnormalities modalities such as HFNO or NIV support may be required, however, patients with severe ARDS may require invasive mechanical ventilation or extracorporeal membrane oxygenation (venovenous ECMO) to maintain adequate gas exchange. Encouraging the non-intubated patients for prone position has been useful in improving the oxygenation if they tolerate proning for more than 3 hours continuously.

Patients with severe ARDS require several maneuvres for recruitment of collapsed alveoli which help in reducing elastance and improve compliance, such as incremental PEEP, other alveolar recruitment maneuvers, along with prone position. Prone positioning promotes alveolar recruitment, reduces ventilation/perfusion mismatch and reduces overinflated area in the lung and thus improves the oxygenation. Prone positioning should always be considered if not contraindicated in patients with PO_2/FiO_2 <150.[6]

The goal of mechanical ventilation in severely hypoxemic patients is to maintain a lung-protective strategy which includes a low tidal volume of 4 to 8 mL/kg predicted body weight (PBW) and restricting plateau pressure below 30 cm H_2O (Fig. 1.1). Two phenotypes of ARDS have been conceptualized in Covid patients, L (Low elastance) type and H (High elastance) type on the basis of responsiveness of PEEP and lung weight on CT scan. The "L type" patients having good pulmonary compliance, can be ventilated with higher tidal volumes (VT) (approximately 7–8 mL/kg of PBW) to avoid absorption atelectasis and hypercapnia. The application of lower PEEP (8–10 cm H_2O) help in preventing the blood flow away from the aerated pulmonary vasculature and thus reduces shunt effect. The H type may progress with worsening of inflammatory edema and self-induced lung injury (P-SILI) may further contribute to worsening. The lung protective ventilation strategy include tidal volume <6 mL/kg and high PEEP with a goal to keep driving pressure below 14 cm H_2O.[7] The prone position and alveolar recruitment strategies may improve oxygenation in refractory cases.

HEMODYNAMIC OPTIMIZATION AND SUPPORT

Myocardial dysfunction with hemodynamic instability is common in critically ill Covid-19 patients. Several factors may contribute including viral toxin, hypoxemia, acute inflammatory responses, increased thrombogenesis, endothelial injury, sympathetic overactivity,

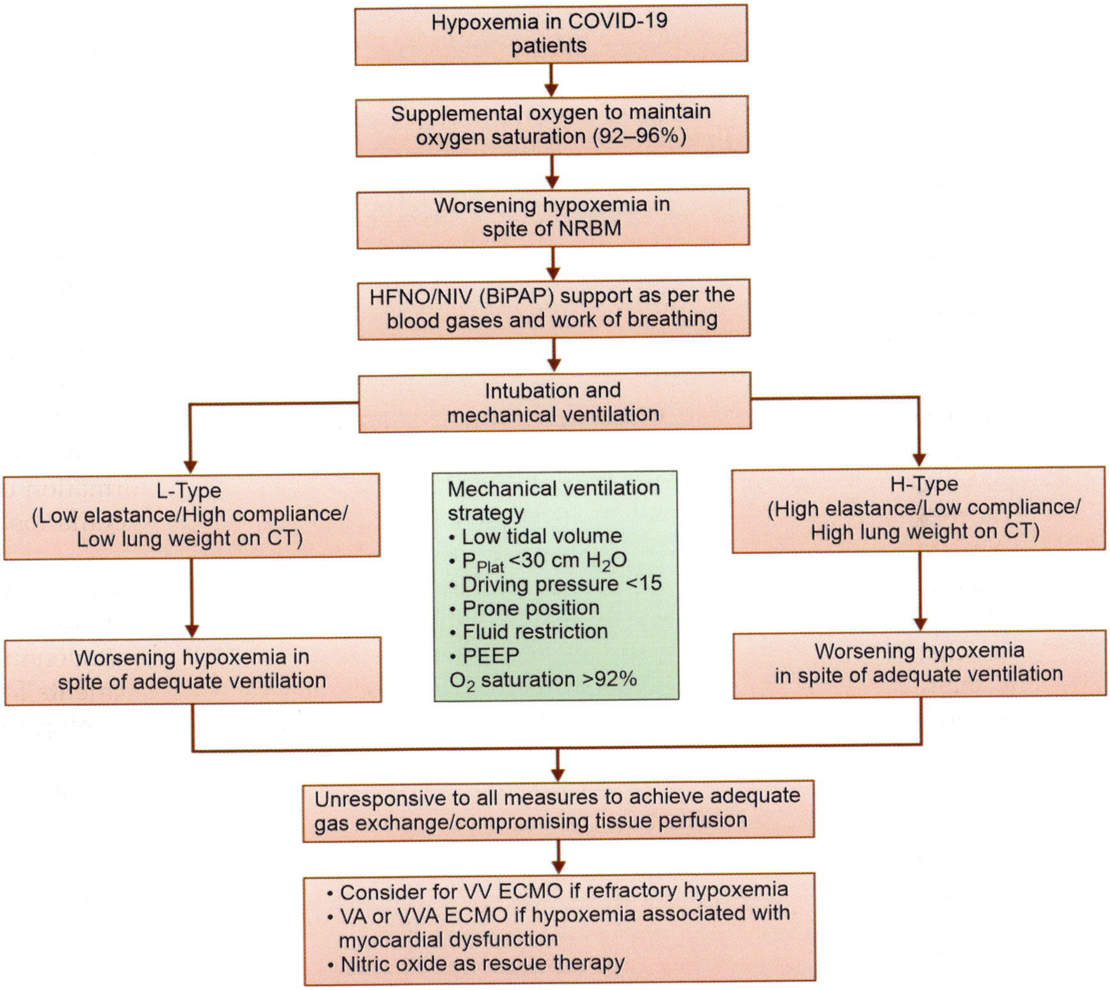

Fig. 1.1: Approach to a hypoxemic Covid-19 patient

myocarditis, vasoconstriction, supply–demand mismatch, poor respiratory reserve, and superadded infections. The various presentations include myocardial injury, arrhythmia, myocarditis with heart failure, arterial or venous thromboembolic event or acute coronary syndrome and cardiogenic shock.[8]

The shock and hemodynamic instability management strategy in severely ill COVID-19 patients include optimizing the blood pressure and cardiac output, thus maintaining tissue perfusion. COVID-induced lung injury and positive pressure ventilation may lead to hemodynamic instability. In addition to COVID-induced pulmonary inflammation, consolidation, microvascular thrombosis and vasoconstriction, hypoxemia and dead space ventilation increases right-ventricular (RV) afterload followed by RV dilatation. The reduction in LV filling due to septal shift may lead to reduction in cardiac output and hemodynamic instability.[9] An optimal fluid balance is important for survival, volume overload is associated with prolonged ICU stay and poor outcome. Whereas hypovolemia may lead to tissue hypoperfusion, thrombus formation and may worsen hypoxemia especially in COVID-19 patients. The various methods for assessment of fluid status include fluid challenge test by administering crystalloid fluid boluses and assess the dynamic indices such as cardiac index and/or velocity–time integral (VTI). The change in pulse pressure variation (PPV) may be assessed by transiently increasing the tidal volume in deeply sedated ARDS patients. Advanced hemodynamic modalities with assessment of dynamic variable may be applied if fluid management is challenging.[10, 11]

COVID-19 induced myocardial depression may occur in severely affected patients and around 1% patients may develop fulminant myocarditis. Troponin levels, natriuretic peptide monitoring and echocardiography assessment may help in early detection of myocardial dysfunction. Echocardiography can be a useful tool in diagnosis and assessment of fluid responsiveness during shock management. If haemodynamic instability persists in spite of adequate fluid administration, norepinephrine infusion should be considered as first-line vasopressor. Norepinephrine infusion may also improve RV function in ARDS patients by improving arterial blood pressure and thus RV blood supply. Vasopressin infusion may be started as second-line vasopressor if adequate blood pressure is not achieved with norepinephrine alone. Dobutamine infusion may be initiated as inotropic agent in case of cardiac dysfunction with acute decompensated heart failure.

Prone positioning should be used in cases of refractory hypoxemia if there is no contraindication. The use of inhaled selective pulmonary vasodilators which help in improving the RV afterload and RV function and thus improve the haemodynamics.

Isolated ARDS or ARDS associated with severe myocardial dysfunction unresponsive to mechanical ventilation and high doses of vasoactive drugs may be considered for VV ECMO (isolated ARDS) or VA ECMO (associated with myocardial dysfunction). However, a hybrid ECMO (V-AV or V-VA) may be required to prevent upper body hypoxemia in worsening of ARDS with VA ECMO.

RENAL DYSFUNCTION AND MANAGEMENT

Besides respiratory failure, the other organ dysfunctions due to COVID-19 include heart and kidney. The incidence of acute kidney injury (AKI) in severe COVID-19 patient is around 6–7% but carries a very high mortality risk especially those patients who are having hematuria or proteinuria, underlying renal dysfunction or AKI as per AKIN (Acute Kidney Injury Network) criteria II or more.[12] COVID-19 associated AKI may occur possibly due to cytokine storm, organ crosstalk or due to infection. Cytokine-induced injury due to release of several mediators IL-6/IL-8/IL-10/IL-18, etc. leading to cytokine storm.[13] This may lead to increased vascular permeability and hypovolemia due to fluid shift and also cause myocardial dysfunction. This may lead to AKI and is labelled as cardiorenal syndrome Type I. Cytokines removal using extracorporeal therapies may be useful in COVID-19 patients who develop acute kidney injury. The other mechanism leading to AKI is organ crosstalk where one injured organ (alveoli in ARDS) may produce tubular injury. Hemodynamic instability may lead to AKI, whereas rhabdomyolysis, metabolic acidosis, and hyperkalemia further worsen the AKI in COVID-19 patients.

The management included the haemodynamic optimization, treatment of sepsis and other supportive measures such as correction of hyperkalemia and metabolic acidosis. The loop diuretics may be used in cases of volume overload. Patients who are unresponsive to medical management should be supported with renal replacement therapy (RRT). The indications for RRT for AKI in critically ill patients are similar in COVID-19 patients. CRRT may be preferred in critically ill patients with potential of haemodynamic instability. However, sustained low-efficiency dialysis (SLED) can also be performed in critically ill patients. The selection of therapy depends upon several factors including cost, expertise and availability of resources as well as reduction of exposure risk. The most common anticoagulation used during CRRT is regional citrate, however, due to risk of circuit thrombosis in COVID-19 patients or if patient is already on heparin, anticoagulation should be achieved with nonfractioned heparin.

METABOLIC DERANGEMENTS

The most common comorbidities encountered during COVID-19 infection are diabetes, hypertension, and cardiovascular diseases (CVD). Patients having diabetic are more often associated with severe COVID-19 infection. Blood sugar monitoring is essential throughout the ICU course, especially those patients who are receiving steroid. The poor blood sugar management is associated with increased morbidity and mortality (Table 1.1).[14]

Table 1.1: Blood glucose management
Regular monitoring of blood glucose level in severe COVID-19 patients
Maintaining pH, electrolytes and checking plasma glucose level
Use of intravenous insulin infusion in severe COVID-19 cases (ARDS and shock) to achieve adequate glycemic control Target blood glucose level: 110–180 mg%

OTHER MANAGEMENT

Remdesivir is most important antiviral therapy at present in severe Covid-19 infection. This is basically a prodrug and inhibits viral RNA polymerases after metabolizing to an analogue of adenosine triphosphate. The use of Remdesivir is associated with reduced mortality and length of hospital stay. The drug is administered intravenously (200 mg IV on day one and 100 mg IV daily 5–10 days). Recently the combination of lopinavir/ritonavir alongwith interferon beta-1b and ribavirin has shown reduced hospital stay and clinical improvement in severely ill COVID-19 patients.[15]

Corticosteroids have shown mortality benefit in COVID-19 patients requiring oxygen or mechanical ventilation. The dose of steroids in COVID-19:[16]

- Methylprednisolone 0.5 mg/kg I/V twice a day for 5 days or
- Dexamethasone 6 mg I/V once daily for 10 days or
- Dexamethasone 20 mg I/V once daily for 5 days and then 10 mg once daily for next 5 days.

Drugs with **Immunomodulation** potential such as tocilizumab, sarilumab, anakinra, reparixin, interferon-α etc. have been used for improving outcomes in COVID-19 patients. Tocilizumab administration has shown the reduction in mechanical ventilation days and decrease in serum IL-6 level. The maximum benefits may be achieved with the early use of Tocilizumab in ICU patients prior to intubation. This potential benefit is possibly related to high levels of IL-6, D-dimer, C-reactive protein, LDH, and ferritin.[17] However, recent randomized trial did not support the benefit with the use of tocilizumab in COVID-19 patients.

ANTICOAGULATION MANAGEMENT

COVID-19 infection induces the thromboinflammatory response with thrombus formation due to multiple factors such as endothelial damage, inflammation, inappropriate fibrinolysis, reduction of natural anticoagulants, and activation of coagulation factors. These patients have higher incidence of deep venous thrombosis and pulmonary embolism. So pharmacologic venous thromboembolism (VTE) prophylaxis should be used in all hospitalized COVID-19 patients if not contraindicated.[18] The anticoagulation regimens may be modified in obese patients, patients with severe thrombocytopenia or deteriorating renal function. What remains to be confirmed is the real role of therapeutic anticoagulation in these patients. The dose of enoxaparin for therapeutic anticoagulation in high risk category is 1 mg/kg twice daily or unfractionated heparin infusion may be given targeting aPTT 60–80 seconds. In the low risk category group, enoxaparin 40 mg once daily dose should be administered.[19]

REFERENCES

1. Wu Z, McGoogan JM. Characteristics of and important lessons from the Coronavirus Disease 2019 (COVID-19) outbreak in China: Summary of a report of 72314 cases from the Chinese center for disease control and prevention. JAMA. 2020;323(13):1239.
2. Centers for Disease Control and Prevention. Underlying medical conditions associated with higher risk for severe COVID-19: information for healthcare professionals. 2022. Available at: https://www.cdc.gov/coronavirus/2019-ncov/hcp/clinical-care/underlyingconditions.html
3. Malik P, Patel U, Mehta D, Patel N, Kelkar R, Akrmah M, et al. Biomarkers and outcomes of COVID-19 hospitalisations: systematic review and meta-analysis. BMJ Evid Based Med. 2021;26:107–108.
4. Fanelli V, Vlachou A, Ghannadian S, Simonetti U, Slutsky AS, Zhang H. Acute respiratory distress syndrome: new definition, current and future therapeutic options. J Thorac Dis. 2013 Jun;5(3):326–34.
5. Diehl JL, Peron N, Chocron R, Debuc B, Guerot E, Hauw-Berlemont C, et al. Respiratory mechanics and gas exchanges in the early course of COVID-19 ARDS: a hypothesis-generating study. Ann Intensive Care. 2020;10(1):95.
6. Shelhamer M, Wesson PD, Solari IL, Jensen DL, etal. Prone Positioning in Moderate to Severe Acute Respiratory Distress Syndrome due to COVID-19: A Cohort Study and Analysis of Physiology. J Intensive Care Med. 2021;36(2):241–52.
7. Sorbello M, El-Boghdadly K, Di Giacinto I, Cataldo R, Esposito C, Falcetta S, et al. The Italian coronavirus disease 2019 outbreak: recommendations from clinical practice. Anaesthesia. 2020;75(6):724–32
8. Costa I, Bittar CS, Rizk SI, Araújo Filho AE, Santos KAQ, Machado TIV, et al. The heart and COVID-19: what cardiologists need to know. Arq Bras Cardiol. 2020;114(5):805–16.
9. Vieillard-Baron A, Matthay M, Teboul JL, Bein T, Schultz M, Magder S, et al. Experts' opinion on management of hemodynamics in ARDS patients: focus on the effects of mechanical ventilation. Intensive Care Med. 2016;42(5):739–49.
10. Kang Y, Chen T, Mui D, Ferrari V, Jagasia D, Scherrer-Crosbie M, et al. Cardiovascular manifestations and treatment considerations in covid-19. Heart. 2020;106(15):1132–41.
11. Malbrain M, Van Regenmortel N, Saugel B, De Tavernier B, Van Gaal PJ, Joannes-Boyau O, et al. Principles of fluid management and stewardship in septic shock: it is time to consider the four D's and the four phases of fluid therapy. Ann Intensive Care. 2018;8(1):66.
12. Cheng Y, Luo R, Wang K, Zhang M, Wang Z, Dong L, et al. Kidney disease is associated with in-hospital death of patients with COVID-19. Kidney Int. 2020;97(5):829–38.
13. Panitchote A, Mehkri O, Hastings A, Hanane T, Demirjian S, Torbic H, et al. Factors associated with acute kidney injury in acute respiratory distress syndrome. Ann Intensive Care. 2019;9(1):74.
14. Yang JK, Feng Y, Yuan MY, Yuan SY, Fu HJ, Wu BY, et al. Plasma glucose levels and diabetes are independent predictors for mortality and morbidity in patients with SARS. Diabet Med. 2006;23(6):623–8.
15. Sheahan TP, Sims AC, Leist SR, Schäfer A, Won J, Brown AJ, et al. Comparative therapeutic efficacy of remdesivir and combination lopinavir, ritonavir, and interferon beta against MERS-CoV. Nat Commun. 2020;11(1):222.
16. Tomazini BM, Maia IS, Cavalcanti AB, Berwanger O, Rosa RG, Veiga VC, et al. Effect of dexamethasone on days alive and ventilator-free in patients with moderate or severe acute respiratory distress syndrome and COVID-19: the CoDEX Randomized Clinical Trial. JAMA. 2020;324(13):1307–16.
17. Xu X, Han M, Li T, Sun W, Wang D, Fu B, et al. Effective treatment of severe COVID-19 patients with tocilizumab. Proc Natl Acad Sci USA. 2020;117(20):10970–5.
18. Maatman TK, Jalali F, Feizpour C, Douglas A 2nd, McGuire SP, Kinnaman G, et al. Routine venous thromboembolism prophylaxis may be inadequate in the hypercoagulable state of severe Coronavirus Disease 2019. Crit Care Med. 2020.
19. Cui S, Chen S, Li X, Liu S, Wang F. Prevalence of venous thromboembolism in patients with severe novel coronavirus pneumonia. J Thromb Haemost. 2020;18(6):1421–4.

CHAPTER

2

Intensive Care Management of Acute Heart Failure

Lilanthi Subasinghe

CASE PRESENTATION

A 62-year-old woman with a history of type 2 diabetes mellitus and hypertension presented with one week history of worsening exertional chest pain and dyspnoea. She denied any fever, cough or wheeze. At the time of presentation, she was conscious and rational. Her peripheries were cold, respiratory rate was 40 breaths per minute and her oxygen saturation (SpO_2) was 90% on room air. She had a heart rate of 128 beats per minute and her blood pressure was 98/60. Lungs revealed bi-basal fine crepitations. The 12-lead electrocardiogram (ECG) showed ST depressions and T inversions in anterolateral leads, troponin I level was 0.8 ng/mL (0–0.04 ng/mL), while liver and functions were within normal range. Her chest X-ray (CXR) is shown in Fig. 2.1. Bedside echocardiogram showed hypokinesia involving the anterior and lateral walls and septum, with left ventricular ejection fraction (LVEF) of 30–35%. She was given the loading doses of antiplatelets and statin and was started on an intravenous (IV) frusemide infusion followed by subcutaneous enoxaparin 1 mg/kg twice daily. Her oxygenation progressively deteriorated and ultimately was started on non-invasive ventilation (CPAP) with pressure support (PS) of 10 cm H_2O and positive end expiratory pressure (PEEP) of 8 cm H_2O. She became progressively hypotensive needing close hemodynamic monitoring and support.

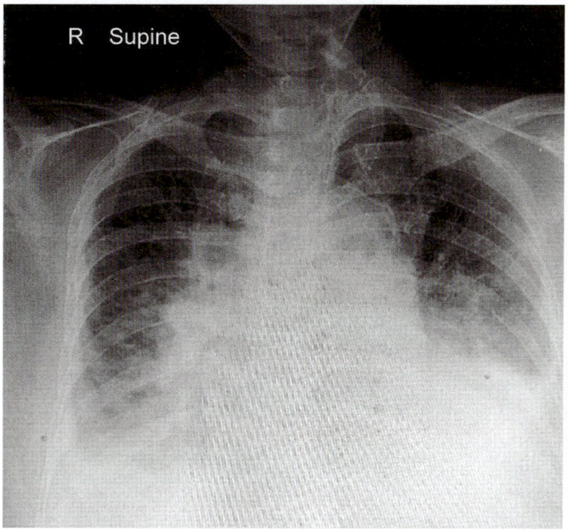

Fig. 2.1: Chest X-ray

How would you Improve this Patient's Haemodynamic Instability?

Vasoactive agents and close hemodynamic monitoring: Her vital parameters were regularly monitored and continued on CPAP. Serial arterial blood gases were carried out to assess oxygenation, acid–base balance and lactate levels. Adequate arterial oxygenation was maintained on the above CPAP settings throughout the stay and she avoided the need for invasive ventilation. Invasive arterial blood pressure monitoring was established with a defined mean arterial pressure (MAP) target of 70–80 mmHg. She was started on

IV noradrenaline infusion titrated according to the target MAP. She was continued on IV frusemide infusion which was titrated and weaned according to the diuresis and lung decongestion. She was started on dual antiplatelet therapy and statin along with enoxaparin. Fluid intake was restricted to 1.5–1.8 litres initially which was gradually increased as she recovered, to 2.4 litres a day. Her electrolyte balance was looked into as well as the blood sugar control was achieved with basal-bolus insulin regime. The course was not complicated with any other organ failures and her inflammatory markers were within normal range. She made an uneventful recovery with gradual weaning from CPAP and noradrenaline. Subsequently she was stabilised on long term heart failure medications along with antiplatelets. She was planned for an interval coronary angiography and was discharged to the cardiology follow up.

PRINCIPLES OF MANAGEMENT

Diagnosis

Heart failure (HF) is defined as inability to deliver oxygen in sufficient amounts to metabolising tissues, resulting from an abnormality of the structure and function of the heart. When there is rapid onset of symptoms and signs of HF, needing urgent interventions, it is called acute heart failure (AHF). The diagnosis of AHF can be challenging, especially in older populations, due to the similarity of AHF symptoms with other respiratory comorbidities like chronic obstructing pulmonary disease (COPD), bronchial asthma (BA) and pneumonia.[1,2] Symptoms and signs of HF result from congestion due to elevated filling pressures, of left (dyspnoea, orthopnoea, paroxysmal nocturnal dyspnoea, lung crepitations, hypoxia, noticeable S3, loud P2 and murmurs) or right (systemic congestion resulting in oedema in dependent regions, hepatic congestion with tender hepatomegaly, congestion in kidneys, intestine and lower extremities, ascites, high jugular venous pressure) side of the heart or both. Any type of HF can give rise to symptoms and signs attributable to low cardiac output states, including cold extremities, hypotension, narrow pulse pressure, pulses alternans and oliguria. The diagnosis of AHF is further supported by advanced haemodynamic parameters monitored via pulse contour analysis combined with either transpulmonary thermodilution (PiCCO) or bolus indicator dilution (LiDCO) methods.[1,2,3] Pulmonary artery catheterisation (PAC) studies can be very useful in properly selected patients, especially with unclear aetiology.[3]

Aetiologies and Precipitating Factors

The commonest etiologies for AHF include ischaemia, inflammation, arrhythmia and acute valve insufficiency. Decompensation of existing HF can occur without a clear precipitant, and also with any of the causes above plus infection, uncontrolled hypertension and non-compliance (Table 2.1). Among the causes which need urgent attention and treatment include, acute ***C***oronary syndromes (ACS), ***H***ypertensive emergency, unstable ***A***rrhythmias, acute ***M***echanical causes, ***P***ulmonary embolism, ***I***nfection and ***T***amponade (Acronym: ***CHAMPIT***).[1,3,4] Patients with AHF commonly have other co-existing co-morbidities (e.g. Type II Diabetes mellitus, atherosclerosis, renovascular disease, anaemia, obstructive sleep apnoea) which may contribute to the pathology, thus need to be considered as therapeutic targets.

Investigations

ECG is essential to exclude ischaemia and arrhythmias. CXR will give evidence of pulmonary oedema and other comorbidities which will present in a similar way as AHF. Radiological

Table 2.1: Aetiological factors triggering AHF	
Precipitants of rapid decompensation	***Precipitants of slower decompensation***
ACS	Non-compliance with diuretics and fluid restriction
Complications of ACS	Infection
E.g.: Ruptures intraventicular septum/papillary muscle/Chordae of mitral valve	
RV infarction	Anaemia
Tachyarrhythmias or severe bradyarrhythmias	Worsening pre-existing valvular dysfunction
Pulmonary embolism	Severe thyroid dysfunction
Cardiac tamponade	Exacerbation of lung disease: Chronic obstructive pulmonary disease
Aortic dissection	Renal failure
Hypertensive crisis	Hypertension
Peripartum cardiomyopathy	Iatrogenic–NSAIDs, steroids
Cerebrovascular insult (neurogenic pulmonary oedema)	Metabolic/hormonal derangements

evidence of pulmonary venous congestion, interstitial oedema and cardiomegaly suggest AHF. Full blood count, urine full report, blood urea, serum creatinine, serum electrolytes and troponin levels detect precipitants of decompensation.[1,2] The B-type natriuretic peptide (BNP) and N-terminal-proBNP (NT-proBNP) are useful in the diagnosis of AHF. A BNP level less than 100 pg/mL strongly suggests non-heart failure aetiology for dyspnoea, greater than 400 pg/mL strongly suggests AHF, while a BNP level between 100–400 pg/mL is considered indeterminate.[3] Ultrasound imaging of the lungs aids in identifying evidence of pulmonary oedema ("B" profile). Doppler echocardiography is the most useful non-invasive modality of imaging in AHF, providing information on cardiac structure and function. Relative wall motion abnormalities and estimates of haemodynamics help in the management.[1,3] Arterial blood gas analysis is handy in evaluating acid–base and lactate status, to assess the response to treatment.

Clinical Classification of AHF

The clinical classification is based on the presence or absence of congestion ("wet" *vs* "dry") and/or the presence or absence of hypoperfusion ("cold" *vs* "warm").[3,4,5] The combinations of these findings define 4 major clinical categories with possible overlaps between them (Table 2.2). These clinical entities require different treatments.

Initial Management

a. Goals of Management

Immediate aim of management is to improve symptoms by restoring oxygenation and improving organ perfusion (Fig. 2.2), simultaneously avoiding cardiac, renal and other organ damage as well. One should consider life-saving therapies, including mechanical circulatory support (MCS) to stabilise the patient and optimize treatment. Following acute management, treatment should be targeted to prevent early readmission and to improve symptoms and survival.

Table 2.2: Clinical presentations of acute heart failure

	Acute decompensated heart failure	*Acute pulmonary oedema*	*Isolated right ventricular failure*	*Cardiogenic shock*
Main mechanisms	LV dysfunction Sodium and water renal retention	Increased afterload and/or predominant LV diastolic dysfunction Valvular heart disease	RV dysfunction and/or pre-capillary pulmonary hypertension	Severe cardiac dysfunction
Main cause of symptoms	Fluid accumulation, increased intraventricular pressure	Fluid redistribution to the lungs and acute respiratory failure	Increased central venous pressure and often systemic hypoperfusion	Systemic hypoperfusion
Onset	Gradual (days)	Rapid (hours)	Gradual or rapid	Gradual or rapid
Main haemodynamic abnormalities	Increased LVEDP and PCWP[a] Low or normal cardiac output Normal to low SBP	Increased LVEDP and PCWP[a] Normal cardiac output Normal to high SBP	Increased RVEDP Low cardiac output Low SBP	Increased LVEDP and PCWP[a] Low cardiac output Low SBP
Main clinical presentations	Wet and warm or Dry and cold	Wet and warm[b]	Dry and cold or Wet and cold	Wet and cold
Main treatment	Diuretics Inotropic agent/ vasopressors (if peripheral hypoperfusion/ hypotension) Short-term MCS or RRT, if needed	Diuretics Vasodilators[b]	Diuretics for peripheral congestion Inotropic agents/ vasopressors (if peripheral hypoperfusion/ hypotension) Short-term MCS or RRT if needed	Inotropic agents/ vasopressors Short-term MCS RRT

LV = Left ventricular; LVEDP = Left ventricular end-diastolic pressure; MCS = Mechanical circulatory support; PCWP = Pulmonary capillary wedge pressure; RV = Right ventricular; RVEDP = Right ventricular end-diastolic pressure; RRT = Renal replacement therapy; SBP = Systolic blood pressure.

[a]May be normal with low cardiac output.

[b]Wet and cold profile with need of inotropes and/or vasopressors may rarely occur.

The process of management needs an integrative approach where continuous assessment and treatment are provided within a shorter time frame. A suggested framework for the early phase management of AHF and associated cardiogenic shock are demonstrated in Figs 2.3 and 2.4.

b. Oxygen Therapy and Ventilatory Support

Correction of hypoxia is critical as hypoxia (and hypercarbia) observed in patients with pulmonary congestion, has negative effects on coronary and pulmonary perfusion. Administration of oxygen should be reserved for hypoxic patients with SpO_2 <90% or partial

Acute cardiac decompensation	
Therapeutic goals	• Restoration of organ perfusion • Weaning of vasoactive drugs • Avoid complications of disease and treatment • Planning of specific intervention(s) • Establish treatment goals - Recovery, Bridge, Palliation
Respiratory support	Aim: Correction of life-threatening hypoxia • Airway management • Oxygen delivery • CPAP/NIPPV • IPV
Haemodynamic assessment	Aim: Assessment of severity of compromise • Examination • ABG (Lactate) and blood to assess organ injury • Echocardiography • CO monitoring
Haemodynamic stabilization	Aim: Organ and tissue perfusion • Optimization of preload, afterload and CO • Commence vasoactive agents • Correction of ischaemia, arrhythmias and specific triggers
Causative etiology	Aim: Identify cause of decompensation • Diagnostic work up using CHAMP • Aetiological specific interventions • Cardiology specialty input • Consider transfer to specialist centre
Progressive or refractory shock	Aim: Establish escalation strategy • MDT/shock team involvement • Consider short team MCS • Assess eligibility for durable MCS or transplantation • Palliation

Fig. 2.2: Management principles of acute cardiogenic shock

ABG, Arterial blood gas; CHAMP, acute Coronary syndrome, Hypertension emergency, Arrhythmia, acute Mechanical cause, Pulmonary embolism; CO, cardiac output; CPAP, continuous positive airway pressure; MCS, mechanical circulatory support; MDT, multidisciplinary team; NIPPV, non-invasive positive-pressure ventilation; IPPV, invasive positive pressure ventilation

pressure of oxygen (PaO_2) < 8.0 kPa (60 mmHg).[4] The use of non-invasive positive pressure ventilation (NIPPV) in the form of continuous (CPAP) or Bi-level (BiPAP) positive airway pressure, helps in alveolar recruitment, redistribution of extravascular lung water, and in improving compliance and surfactant production, thus reducing the shunt and work of breathing.[5] Use of NIPPV needs to be used in patients with respiratory distress as evidenced by tachypnoea (respiratory rate >25 breaths/min) and desaturation (SpO_2 <90%). It should be instigated immediately to alleviate symptoms, to reduce the rate of invasive ventilation and hospital mortality[4,5] paying careful attention to avoid hypotension. Invasive positive pressure ventilation (IPPV) is indicated, if there is respiratory failure leading to hypoxaemia (PaO_2 <60 mmHg), hypercapnia ($PaCO_2$ >50 mmHg) and acidosis (pH <7.35), which cannot be managed non-invasively. PPV reduces pulmonary wedge pressure, LV afterload, myocardial oxygen demand and work of breathing, thus improves cardiac index and oxygenation.

c. Cardiovascular Management

One main target in managing AHF patients is to restore adequate cardiac output aiming to establish adequate tissue perfusion to prevent end organ damage. Specific precipitants

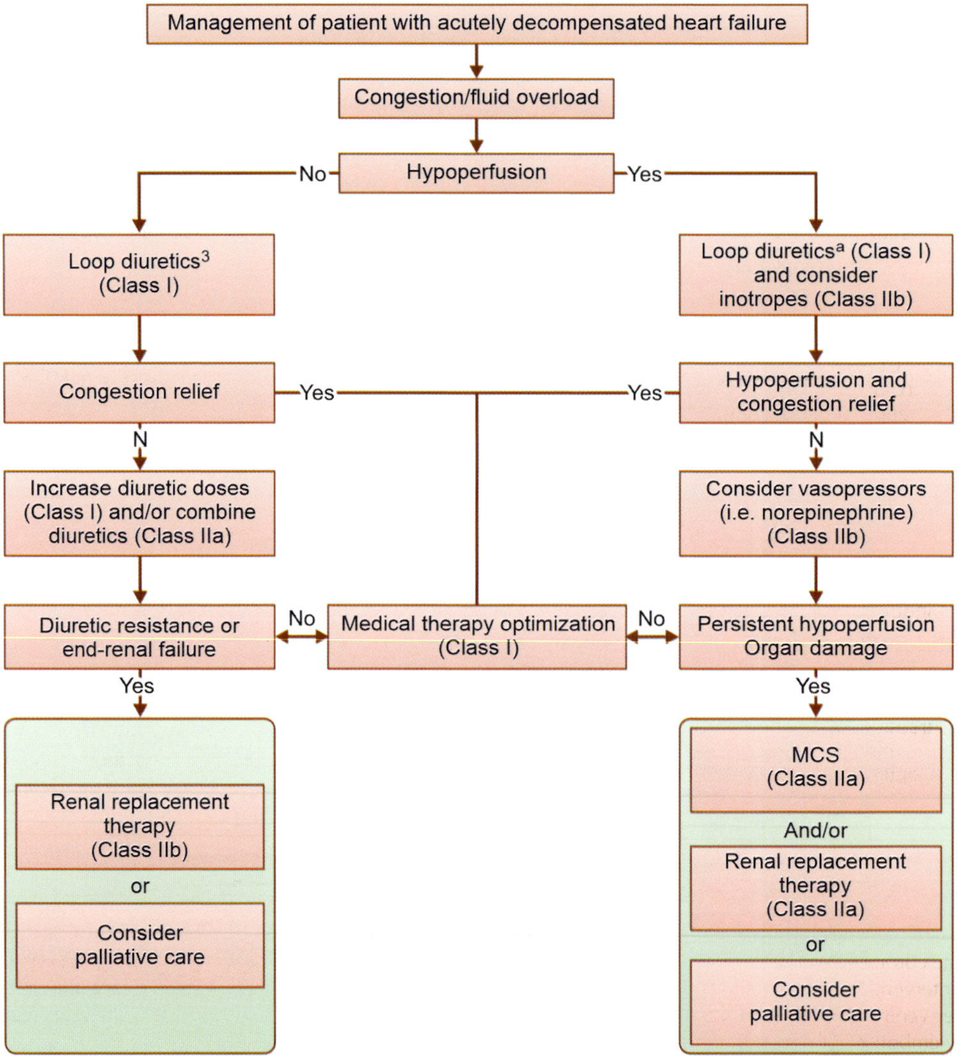

Fig. 2.3: Management of acute decompensated heart failure

MCS = Mechanical circulatory support. [a]Adequate diuretic doses to relieve congestion and close monitoring of diuresis is recommended regardless of perfusion status.

(Re-use permission obtained from the publisher)

need to be managed as they are diagnosed, e.g. referring for coronary angiography within the first 120 minutes with an intent to achieve complete revascularisation, in acute coronary syndromes (ACS).[4,5] Diuretics (mainly loop diuretics) play a major role in alleviating symptoms and signs of fluid overload by dual action of diuresis and vasodilation. To start with intravenous diuretics and vasodilators are indicted to relieve dyspnoea, titrated to blood pressure (BP). Intravenous furosemide is used most commonly as the first-line diuretic. One should use the lowest dose possible to provide adequate clinical effect and should be modified according to patients renal function.[4] Attention should be paid to avoid hypokalaemia, renal impairment and hypovolaemia. Intravenous vasodilators (Table 2.3) are also used in AHF for symptomatic relief; however, there is no robust evidence confirming their beneficial effects. Opioid agents have both anxiolytic action and vasodilatory effects in the setting of acute

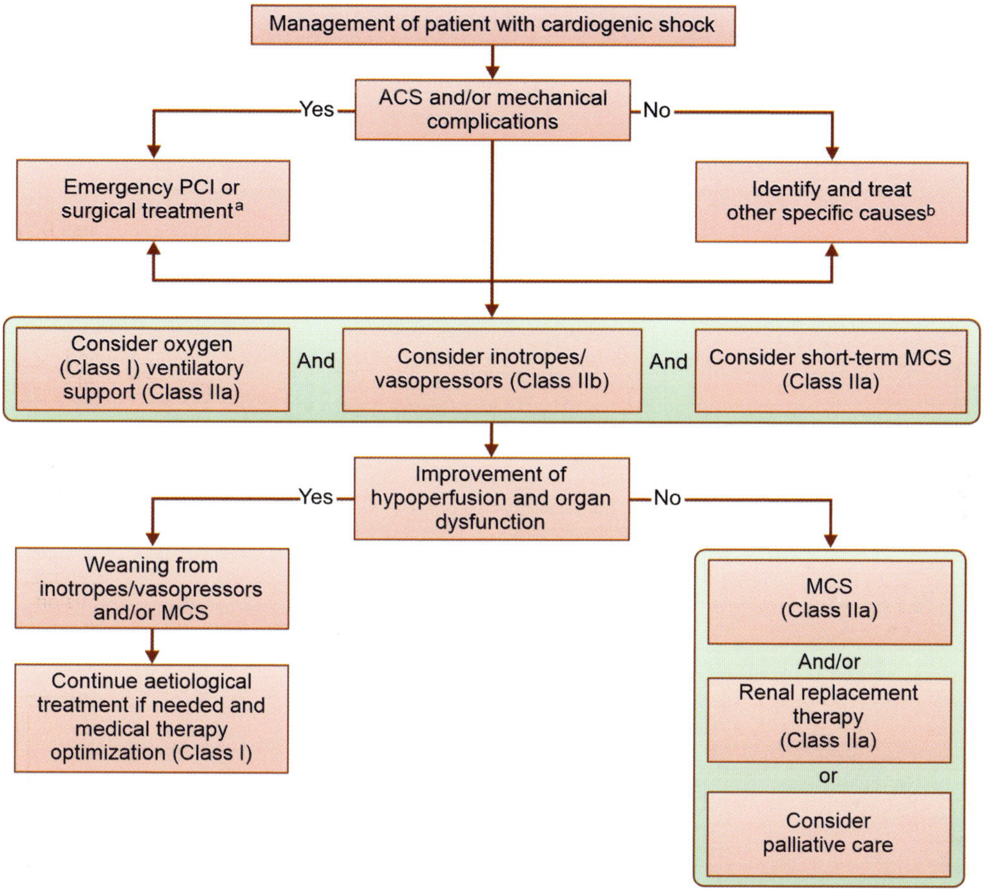

Fig. 2.4: Management of cardiogenic shock

ACS = Acute coronary syndrome; BTT = Bridge to transplantation; MCS = Mechanical circulatory support; PCI = Percutaneous coronary intervention. [a]PCI in ACS, pericardiocentesis in tamponade, mitral valve surgery in papillary muscle rupture. In case of inter-ventricular septum rupture, MCS as BTT should be considered. [b]Other causes include acute valve regurgitation, pulmonary embolism, infection, acute myocarditis, arrhythmia

(Re-use permission obtained from the publisher)

Table 2.3: Intravenous vasodilators used to treat acute heart failure

Vasodilator	*Dosing*	*Main side effects*	*Other*
Nitroglycerine	Start with 10–20 μg/min, increase up to 200 μg/min	Hypotension, headache	Tolerance on continuous use
Isosorbide dinitrate	Start with 1 mg/h, increase up to 10 mg/h	Hypotension, headache	Tolerance on continuous use
Nitroprusside	Start with 0.3 μg/kg/min and increase up to 5 μg/kg/min	Hypotension, isocyanate toxicity	Light sensitive

pulmonary oedema. However, they can cause respiratory depression and potentiate the need for invasive ventilation. Their use is not routine and should be considered cautiously.[4] Furthermore, prompt correction of acidosis, optimisation of cardiac preload with balanced crystalloid challenges where clinically indicated and optimising afterload, need to be given

Table 2.4: Summary of the effects of positive inotropes and/or vasopressors used to treat acute heart failure

Medication	*Bolus dose*	*Infusion* *Rate 0.05–0.5 μg/kg/min unless stated*	*Effect*	*Receptors*				
				Alpha 1	*Beta 1*	*Beta 2*	*Dopamine*	*V1*
Catecholamines								
Epinephrine	Bolus: 1 mg can be given IV during resuscitation, repeated every 3–5 min	0.01–0.1 0.1–0.5	↑ SVR, ↑↑ CO ↑↑ SVR, ↑ CO					
Norepinephrine	No	0.2–1.0	↑↑ SVR, ↑ CO					
Dopamine	No	0.5–2 5–10 >10	↑ CO ↑↑ CO, ↑ SVR ↑↑ SVR, ↑ CO	 + +++	+ +++ ++	 + 	+++ ++ ++	
Dobutamine	No	2–20	↑↑ CO, ↓ SVR, ↓ PVR	+	++++	++		
Phosphodiesterase inhibitors								
Milrinone	25–75 μg/kg over 10–20 min	0.375–0.75	↑ CO, ↓ SVR, ↓ PVR					
Calcium sensitisers								
Levosimendan	12 μg/kg over 10 min (optional)	0.1, which can be decreased to 0.05 or increased to 0.2	↑ CO, ↓ SVR, ↓ PVR					
Vasoconstrictors								
Phenylephrine		0.1–10	↑↑ SVR	++++				
Vasopressin	No	0.02–0.04 U/min	↑↑ SVR ↔ PVR					++++

↑, Increase; ↑↑, Significant increase; ↓, Decrease; ↔, No effect or modest decrease; +, Increase

CO, cardiac output; PVR, peripheral vascular resistance; SVR, systemic vascular resistance; V1, vasopressin one receptor.

due attention. Vasoactive agents play a major role in improving organ perfusion (Table 2.4). Nonetheless, there is scarcity of good quality evidence, on which no firm recommendations on the first choice of vasopressor or inotrope can be drawn.[6,7] All efforts should be made to select the agent according to the clinical need and to minimise the number of agents and their doses. In summary, inotropes increase the cardiac contractility at the expense of increased heart rate (HR), thus myocardial oxygen demand by compromising diastolic filling, reducing CO as well the coronary perfusion time leading to myocardial ischaemia, whereas vasopressors counteract vasodilation which in turn will increase the afterload and cardiac work. The choice of the vasoactive agent with supportive evidence is discussed in this section.[1,3]

Further treatment of AHF in shock is guided by haemodynamics parameters. Rough guide would be patients systolic blood pressure (SBP). In cases where SBP is more than 110 mmHg, vasodilator therapy is considered, e.g. intravenous nitrate, reducing the preload and afterload, thereby increasing stroke volume (SV). This is contraindicated in fixed output/afterload dependent states like aortic stenosis, mitral stenosis or hypertrophic cardiomyopathy (HCM) with severe outflow tract obstruction. In patients with SBP less than 90 mmHg, vasoactive agents should be considered. The assessment of response to any haemodynamic support should be done serially with a combination of clinical assessment, biochemical parameters [lactate, central venous oxygen saturations ($ScvO_2$)] and continuous monitoring of haemodynamic variables (echocardiography, CO, cardiac index, PCWP, etc.). This aids in early identification of clinical changes and in titrating pharmacological and device therapy. Central venous cannulation helps in safer administration of vasoactive agents, allows monitoring of central venous pressures and determining $ScvO_2$ as a surrogate marker of tissue oxygen delivery and utilisation. Invasive BP monitoring with arterial catheter and continuous ECG monitoring should be done at a minimum and continuous CO monitoring should be considered wherever feasible. Pulmonary artery catheterisation (PAC) studies should be carried out in selected patients and can be useful in guiding therapy. Weaning of vasoactive support should be initiated once haemodynamic stabilisation is achieved.

d. Mechanical Circulatory Support (Mechanical Assist Devices)

Short-term MCSs, including percutaneous cardiac support devices, extracorporeal life support (ECLS) and extracorporeal membrane oxygenation (ECMO) may be used to support patients with left or biventricular failure as a 'bridge to decision' (BTD). This byes time to stabilize haemodynamics, recover end-organ function and to allow for a complete clinical evaluation for either cardiac transplant or a more durable MCS device.[4,8,9] The use of these devices is restricted to a shorter duration. There is no good evidence that an IABP is of benefit in other causes of cardiogenic shock.[4]

e. Other Considerations in the ICU

i. Sedation: Usually a combination of an opiate (fentanyl, morphine) and a hypnotic (propofol, midazolam) is titrated according to the established sedation scales. Propofol can cause significant hypotension especially in HCM. Alpha agonists like dexmedetomidine and clonidine can cause clinically significant bradycardia and hypotension at low doses and hypertension in higher doses, thus warrants careful usage in AHF.[5]

ii. Renal support: Acute kidney injury (AKI) is seen in about 25% of patients in AHF. It is associated with a poor outcome. Pathophysiology of AKI in AHF is multifactorial and includes venous congestion secondary to right heart failure, reduced renal perfusion pressure due to low CO and usage of nephrotoxic agents. Management of AKI in this setting is largely supportive. The optimal timing of initiation of renal replacement therapy (RRT) is not defined, except for clear indications. Ultrafiltration should be confined to patients with fluid overload who fail to respond to diuretic-based strategies.[5] Initiation of RRT should be reserved for following indications in patients with refractory volume overload: Severe hyperkalaemia (K+ >6.5 mmol/L), severe acidaemia (pH <7.2) and serum urea level >25 mmol/L (150 mg/dL).[4]

iii. Thromboprophylaxis: Thrombo-prophylactic therapy with an anticoagulant (heparin or other) is recommended unless contraindicated otherwise.

f. Management of Specific Situations

i. Acute coronary syndromes: All patients with ST elevation myocardial infarction (STEMI) or new onset left bundle branch block (LBBB) need emergency primary percutaneous coronary intervention (PCI) with an aim of complete revascularisation. Patients with non-ST elevation myocardial infarcts will need urgent revascularisation and depending on the findings might need coronary artery bypass grafting.

ii. Isolated right ventricular infarction: RV infarcts present with elevated right heart pressures, severe tricuspid regurgitation and reduced CO. The common reasons are obstructed right coronary artery or a dominant left circumflex artery or a massive pulmonary embolus. In these patients, diuretics and vasodilators should be used with caution and fluid challenge plays a major role at the outset.

iii. Arrhythmias: When a tachyarrhythmia occurs in the light of AHF it is considered unstable and is managed with synchronised electrical cardioversion. Commonest tachyarrhythmia in this setting is considered to be atrial fibrillation (AF). Stable AF warrants rate control ideally with a beta blocker (BB) in HF. In AHF BB should only be used when the patient is stabilised BP-wise. If with reduced EF, digoxin or amiodarone are the choices. If AHF is with preserved EF, verapamil is an option. Ventricular tachycardia and fibrillation are managed according to the advanced life support algorithm with cardioversion when indicated and with amiodarone. Resistant arrhythmias might need catheter ablation. Implantable cardioverter-defibrillator (ICD) should be considered on discharge. Severe bradycardia and high degree atrio-ventricular blocks need emergency pacing, if associated with AHF.

iv. Valvular problems/acute mechanical cause: Aortic stenosis patients in AHF need surgical evaluation for possible valve replacement, transcatheter valve implantation or balloon valvuloplasty. Vasodilators should be avoided in the management. Mitral stenosis complicated with AHF warrants diuretics and BB and surgical options either percutaneous or open. Acute mitral regurgitation and aortic regurgitation with AHF can occur in acute cardiac ischaemia and endocarditis, leading to a surgical emergency.

v. Cardiac tamponade: Commonly occurs in patients with recent history of cardiac surgery or infarction and high index of suspicion is needed for the diagnosis. Pericardial pressures exceed intracardiac pressures impairing diastolic filling, thus reducing CO. Clinical diagnosis is suggested by low CO in the presence of high filling pressures, pulsus paradoxus and electrical alternans, and is confirmed by echocardiography. Immediate management includes intravascular expansion followed by pericardiocentesis.

vi. Hypertensive emergency: Aggressive BP reduction in the range of 25% during the first few hours and cautiously thereafter, should be considered with intravenous vasodilators and loop diuretics.

g. Refractory Patients–Heart Transplant/Palliation

Being considered as the gold standard, cardiac transplant remains a reserved therapeutic option for resistant HF patients. Admission to ICU with acute decompensation acts as a defining trigger for the work up and possible candidates should be discussed early with a transplant centre where facilities and pathway are established. Short term or durable mechanical ventilatory support will be needed to bridge the patient and stabilise until such transfer process occurs. Cardiac patients needing ICU care is associated with poor outcome and higher mortality. Therefore, it is essential to have patient and family centred discussions at the outset to set goals/ceilings of care. Palliative care and end-of-life care pathways and training should be incorporated to intensive care delivery systems to achieve this objective.

h. Post-stabilization

In patients with HF with reduced EF (HFrEF), angiotensin converting enzyme inhibitor or angiotensin receptor blocker needs to be started as soon as possible since they have a positive effect on LV remodelling and long-term mortality benefit. BB need to be started sooner, once the patient no longer requires intravenous diuretics. It adds to the improvement of LVEF and carries mortality benefit. Both should be started in low doses and sequentially up titrated to their evidence-based targets. Mineralocorticoid receptor antagonists (spironolactone and epleronone) in selected patients with low EF, have shown to reduce all-cause mortality, sudden cardiac death and hospitalisation rates. Ivabradine is used to lower the sinus tachycardia, without affecting the BP, when BBs are contraindicated or cannot be sufficiently titrated. Digoxin is a choice in AF when BB titration is limited. In contrast, long term management of HFpEF has less therapeutic options and includes symptomatic relief with loop diuretics, control of hypertension and arrhythmias.

EVIDENCE CONTOUR

Randomized controlled clinical trials on the use of vasoactive agents (Table 2.5) in cardiogenic shock is limited, and the recommendations are drawn largely from meta-analyses and expert opinions. In the review of existing clinical trials, there remains significant heterogeneity in the literature. Thus, the optimal first-line vasoactive medication in CS remains unclear and no specific drug is recommended unanimously in any cumulative data analyses. The traditional approach was to start on an inotrope, e.g. a non-vasodilatory agent like dobutamine, as the first-line agent. The SOAP II (Sepsis Occurrence in Acutely ill Patients) trial was the largest clinical trial evaluating the use of vasopressors in shock, where dopamine was associated with higher risk of arrhythmias and mortality in cardiogenic shock, thus not recommended routinely.[10] Dobutamine is considered non-inferior to milrinone in cardiogenic shock while levosimendan and milrinone were better in achieving short term outcomes in patients with AHF secondary to acute myocardial infarction.[8]

The majority of culminating new evidence recommends norepinephrine as the primary vasoactive medication of choice, with the subsequent addition of vasopressin to achieve the haemodynamic goal with or without inotropic support.[5,8,9] Further escalation should consider the titrating doses of inotropes, dobutamine, milrinone or levosimendan, cautiously used against the complications of tachyarrhythmias and peripheral vasodilation.[5–8] Nevertheless there is a multitude of studies providing evidence against using darenaline in this setting, as it is observed to produce higher heart rates, higher lactate levels, increased myocardial oxygen

Table 2.5: Landmark RCTs of vasoactive agents

Trial	Year	Intervention	Primary outcome	Secondary outcome	Finding
SOAP	2002	Dopamine *vs* other catecholamines	Increased intensive care mortality Rate with dopamine	—	No difference
RUSSLAN	2002	Levosimendan *vs* placebo	Six hours of levosimendan did not increase hypotension or ischemia significantly	—	Lower with levosimendan
REVIVE-II	2006	Levosimendan *vs* placebo	Reduction in BNP and duration of hospitalization with levosimendan	—	Higher with levosimendan
SURVIVE	2006	Levosimendan *vs* dobutamine	No difference with long outcomes	—	Lower with levosimendan
CATS	2007	Adrenaline *vs* noradrenaline	28-day mortality	Mortality at day 7, 14, 90, ICU/hospital discharge, systemic haemodynamics, arterial pH and, lactate; SOFA, time to haemodynamic success, vasopressor withdrawal	No difference in PO/SO
CAT	2008	Adrenaline *vs* noradrenaline	Achieving MAP goal for >24 h without pressors	28 and 90 days mortality	No difference in PO, SO
VASST	2008	Noradrenaline *vs* vasopressin	28-day mortality	90 days mortality; days alive and free of organ dysfunction, ventilator/ vasopressor/RRT/SIRS/ corticosteroid-free days/ LOS/SAE	No difference in PO/ no difference in SAE
SOAP II	2010	Noradrenaline *vs* dopamine	28-day mortality	ICU, hospital LOS, organ support-free days, time to attainment of haemodynamic stability, changes in haemodynamic variables, use of inotropes	No difference in PO, dopamine associated with more arrhythmias, increased risk of death in cardiogenic shock
LEAF	2014	Levosimendan *vs* placebo	Levosimendan improved contractility in post-ischemic myocardium	—	No difference
VANISH	2016	Noradrenaline *vs* vasopressin	AKI-free days	Mortality, RRT, SAE	No difference in PO, less RRT in vasopressin group
ATHOS 3 group	2017	Angiotensin II *vs* placebo	Predefined increase in MAP at 3 h	Change in SOFA, mortality, change in vasopressor dose	Significantly higher percentage of patients achieving PO. Cardiovascular SOFA significantly lower in treatment
SEPSIS-ACT	2019	Selepressin *vs* placebo	Ventilator- and vasopressor-free days up to day 30	90 days mortality, 30 days ICU, RRT free days	No difference in primary and secondary outcomes

LOS: Length of stay, PO: Primary outcome; RRT: Renal replacement therapy; SAE: Sepsis associated encephalopathy; SIRS: Systemic inflammatory response syndrome; SO: Secondary outcome; SOFA: Sequential organ failure assessment.

demand and increased mortality.[6,7] In a recent meta-analysis, Karami found that treatment with either a vasopressor or an inotrope was not associated with a difference in short-term or long-term mortality, with a positive trend toward better outcome with levosimendan. However, the overall quality of evidence was graded low.[11]

Due to the heterogeneity in the aetiology and triggering factors for CS, some guidelines recommend different vasoactive medications for each presentation of CS. For example, in the management of CS in patients with ST-elevation myocardial infarction norepinephrine is recommended as the vasoconstrictor of choice. To improve cardiac contractility, inotropes like dobutamine may be given simultaneously to norepinephrine.[8] In the light of AHF and CS, the first choice can be shifted to inotropes that would assist in decongestion. Contradictorily, alternative recommendations exist where they suggest inotropes as the first choice (dobutamine and then levosimendan or levosimendan alone as the first), after a thorough assessment of cardiac function and preload optimisation. They advocate that the vasopressors (noradrenaline) should be considered later.[4,7,12]

In conclusion, it is suggested that the approach should be highly individualised by rationalizing and selecting the vasoactive agent depending on the clinical judgement in the given context. Most importantly the patient's clinical response must be monitored and therapy should be guided by a selected strategy of continuous haemodynamic/cardiac output monitoring, especially when a second or third vasoactive medication is required.

CHAPTER

3

Stroke

Gloria Rodríguez-Vega

CASE PRESENTATION

An 80-year-old female with history of hypertension, heart disease, hyperlipidemia, allergic to aspirin and penicillin, who presented at approximately 8:15 am presented with right-sided weakness and inability to talk. Her husband called 9-1-1, took her to the ER where a code stroke was activated. Her initial vital signs were V/S T 36.7 C, P78 bpm, RR 25 bpm BP 175/80 mmHg sats 100%. On examination she was alert, aphasic, mildly dysarthric, but nodded appropriately to simple questions, mild right nasolabial flattening, right-sided hemiparesis. Her National Institutes of Health Stroke Scale (NIHHS) was 10. A head CT scan showed no hemorrhage. After evaluation of inclusion and exclusion criteria, and husband's consent, she was given IV t-PA without improvement of symptoms. Initial glucose 123. Her initial laboratories, including CBC, coagulation panel and BMP were unremarkable. Suspecting large vessel occlusion, a head CT-A was done and revealed a left MCA distal M1 occlusion. Taken to OR for mechanical thrombectomy without complications and successful removal of thrombus after 6 hours of symptoms onset. She was transferred to the neuro-icu awake and extubated, dysarthric and moving all extremities. The rest of her hospital course was uneventful and was later transferred to stroke unit and eventually discharged to an inpatient rehab facility.

What is an Acute Ischemic Stroke?

Introduction

Acute ischemic stroke (AIS) is a treatable medical emergency. It is one of the leading causes of death and a leading cause of long-term disability, medical expenditures and ICU admissions. Gender, age, and race/ethnicity are among non-modifiable risk factors while diabetes mellitus, hypertension, coronary artery disease, atrial fibrillation, hyperlipidemia and smoking are modifiable risk factors. Vascular stenosis, embolic etiologies, hypercoagulable states, and venous hypertension have all been identified as mechanisms for AIS. Goals of care in AIS include restoration of cerebral blood flow and prevention of secondary brain injury.

Clinical Features

AIS is a time sensitive diagnosis that requires high level of suspicion, therefore strong familiarity with common stroke presentation is essential. Clinical presentation is dependent on the vascular territory affected. Sudden onset of neurological signs and symptoms include aphasia, weakness, visual field defects, sensory loss. It is called a transient ischemic attack (TIA) when symptoms resolve within 24 hours. Migraine, hypoglycemia (or other metabolic derangement), sepsis, acute drug intoxication, tumors, Todd's paralysis, and liver failure are other conditions that may mimic a stroke and must be considered in the differential diagnosis. Since this is a clinical and time sensitive diagnosis, whose standard of care includes administering t-PA and excluding hemorrhage with a non-contrast head CT, clinicians must rely on their clinical acumen, standardized stroke assessment tools, such as the NIHSS, and protocols.[1]

Diagnosis

A non-contrast head CT is the most useful test in the management of AIS in most cases. It helps distinguish between hemorrhagic stroke and identifying subtle ischemic changes. MRI diffusion-weighted imaging has a higher sensitivity and specificity for acute infarct than CT.

It is important to determine the mechanism of the acute ischemic stroke. Vascular stenosis, embolic etiologies, hypercoagulable states affecting both venous and arterial circulation and venous hypertension must be investigated to determine the causes of AIS. For this reason, many stroke centers combine CT or MRI imaging with angiography to allow better pathophysiological classification of stroke and therefore implementation of secondary prevention measures.

STANDARD APPROACH TO MANAGEMENT

Acute Management

a. **Airway management:** The airway should be assessed and secured, including intubation for comatose patients. Supplemental oxygen should be given to maintain an oxygen saturation >94%.

b. **Blood pressure:** Except for candidates for IV t-PA whose BP should not exceed 185/110 mmHg hypertension should not be treated acutely after AIS. Lowering blood pressure may affect penumbral perfusion and worsen cerebral ischemia. If a patient develops malignant hypertension BP can be reduced 15% if it exceeds 220/120 mmHg. Antihypertensives medications could be initiated after 24 hours of stroke onset.

c. **Revascularization therapy:** Rapid determination of eligibility for thrombolysis with IV t-PA or mechanical thrombectomy must be made. IV t-PA is considered the standard of care across the world. In the NINDS trial, IV t-PA was shown to be effective at reducing stroke morbidity. (Dose: 0.9 mg/kg, given as a 10% bolus and the remainder in 1 hour.) The benefit of t-PA when given within 3 hours of onset of symptoms is 13% return to baseline function, while 19% have some functional improvement. There is a 6% chance of ICH after t-PA within the 3-hour window. Risk of hemorrhage with reperfusion increases with time. Data from ECASS-III trial supports the use of t-PA within 3-to-4.5-hour window for select patients.[2,3] Hospitals should have protocols with inclusion/exclusion criteria, administration order sets in order to facilitate the safe administration of IV t-PA. If a patient declines during IV t-PA administration, the infusion must be stopped immediately, administer cryoprecipitate, and perform a head CT. Neurosurgical consultation should be requested if intracranial hemorrhage is found. Other complications of IV t-PA administration includes anaphylaxis and angioedema. Treatment includes ranitidine, diphenhydramine, methylprednisolone, and emergent intubation if indicated. Patients should be considered for mechanical thrombectomy within 24 hours (DAWN, DIFFUSE[3]) if there is large vessel occlusion.[4,5] Several open label trials have shown benefit of thrombectomy in addition to IV t-PA or over IV t-PA alone. (MR CLEAN,[6] ESCAPE,[7] SWIFT PRIME,[8] EXTEND-IA,[9] REVASCAT.)[10]

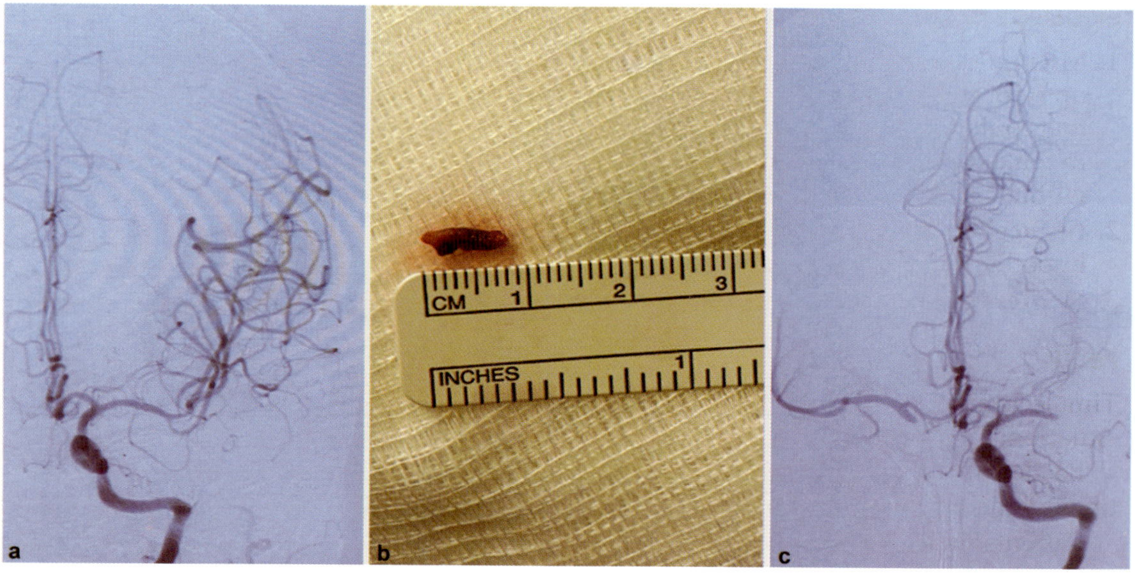

Fig. 3.1: Cerebral angiogram showing left MCA distal M1 occlusion (a) followed by successful removal of clot (b) and follow-up angiogram with revascularization (c) Courtesy of Juan Ramos, MD, neurovascular neurosurgeon.

d. **Malignant hemispheric stroke:** Most commonly defined as middle cerebral artery (MCA) or combined anterior cerebral artery, middle cerebral artery (ACA/MCA) stroke in either hemisphere which involves at least 2/3 territory or is > 100 ml in volume. These strokes have elevated risk for malignant edema and brain herniation.

Medical Management

a. **Cardiac monitoring:** Cardiac arrhythmias, including atrial fibrillation, are common after AIS. Therefore, continuous cardiac monitoring for at least 24 hours is recommended.
b. **Temperature:** Fever suppression is prudent since hyperthermia has been associated with increased mortality in observational studies in humans.[11]
c. **Glucose:** Hypoglycemia worsens cerebral infarction and should be avoided. Guidelines recommended keeping serum glucose between 140–180 mg/dL.[1]
d. **DVT prophylaxis:** DVT prophylaxis should be initiated within 24 hours of hospital admission.
e. **Nutrition:** Since dysphagia is common in AIS patients, assessment of the patient's swallowing ability should be performed and documented in record. Energy demands increase during AIS so early nutrition is important for clinical recovery.
f. **Early mobilization:** Early evaluation by physical and occupational therapy has been shown to improve outcomes.

Secondary Prevention

After diagnosis, treatment and stabilization, implementation of secondary prevention therapies should be implemented. These include the initiation of antiplatelet agents (if no contraindication exists), anticoagulation in patients with atrial fibrillation, management of hypertension and dyslipidemia, screening for diabetes, smoking cessation and carotid revascularization if indicated.

EVIDENCE CONTOUR

1. **MRI guided thrombolysis:** There is a group of acute ischemic stroke patients who wake up with stroke symptoms or had unclear time of onset >4.5 hours from last known well that could be treated with IV alteplase within 4.5 hours of recognition of stroke symptoms. In wake-up trial, MRI was useful for selecting those who can benefit from IV alteplase within 4.5 hours of stroke symptom detection.[12]
2. **Induced hypothermia:** In patients with AIS, the benefit of treatment with induced hypothermia is uncertain.
3. **Depression screening:** Patients should be routinely screened for poststroke depression.[13]

Pearls

Time is brain. Early diagnosis and management of AIS is highly dependent on the clinical situation.

Basilar artery thrombosis. Can mimic seizures with repetitive myoclonic movements, unexplained coma. Look for "dense vessel sign" in head CT.

Patients with improving neurologic signs should still be considered for thrombolysis.

Care of stroke patients in "stroke units" lowers mortality and improves outcomes.

REFERENCES

1. Powers et al. Guidelines for the early management of patients with acute ischemic stroke: 2019 update to the 2018 guidelines for the early management of acute ischemic stroke: A guideline for healthcare professionals from the American Heart Association/American Stroke Association. Stroke 2019;50e344–e418.
2. Cronin et al. Adherence to third European Cooperative Acute Stroke Study 3-to-4.5-hour exclusions and association with outcome: data from Get with the Guidelines-Stroke. Stroke 2014 Sep 45(9):2745–2749.
3. Hacke et al. Thrombolysis with alteplase 3 to 4.5 hours after acute ischemic stroke. N Eng J Med 2008 Sept 25;359 (13) 1317–1329.
4. Nogueria et al. Thrombectomy 6 to 24 Hours after Stroke with a Mismatch between Deficit and Infarct. N Engl J Med 2018;378:11–21.
5. Albers et al. Thrombectomy for Stroke at 6 to 16 Hours with Selection by Perfusion Imaging. N Engl J Med 2018; 378:708–718.
6. Berkhemer et al. A Randomized Trial of Intraarterial Treatment for Acute Ischemic Stroke. N Engl J Med 2015;372:11–20.
7. Goyal et al. Randomized Assessment of Rapid Endovascular Treatment of Ischemic StrokeN Engl J Med 2015;372:1019–30.
8. Saver et al. Stent-Retriever Thrombectomy after Intravenous t-PA vs. t-PA Alone in Stroke. N Engl J Med 2015; 372:2285–2295.
9. Campbell et al. Endovascular Therapy for Ischemic Stroke with Perfusion-Imaging Selection. N Engl J Med 2015; 372:1009–1018.
10. Jovin et al. Thrombectomy within 8 Hours after Symptom Onset in Ischemic Stroke N Engl J Med 2015; 372:2296–2306.
11. Walter et al. The neurological and cognitive consequences of hyperthermia. Critical Care 2016; 20:199.
12. Tomalla et al. MRI-Guided Thrombolysis for Stroke with Unknown Time of Onset. N Engl J Med 2018; 379:611–622.
13. Towfighi et al. Poststroke depression: a scientific statement for healthcare professionals from the American Heart Association/ American Stroke Association. Stroke. 2017;48:e30–e43.

CHAPTER

4

Brain Trauma Injury

Gandra D'Almeida A, Moreno R

CASE PRESENTATION

A 24 years old male, patient arrived to the hospital carried by the extra-hospital emergency services. He is not intubated, having only a Guedel tube and a low-flow oxygen mask; a cervical collar is in place. He has been found inconscient at the bottom of the stairs of his flat. There are no witnesses of the situation, neither any information about previous diseases, namely neurological diseases or drug abuse.

At the observation the patients is in coma (GCS 9: Motor 5, Eyes 3, Verbal 1), without grossly asymmetries in muscular tonus; pupils are in intermediary position, slightly asymmetric, but reactive to light. No tongue biting signs are present. There are two epicraneal hematomas in the skull, without sinking of the cranial cap or crepitation. No otorrhagia was observed. No other grossly lesions were seen in the physical exam, namely on the thorax, abdomen and pelvis. Blood was collected and send to the lab and an exam was asked.

What is the Standard Approach to Management?

As any patient arriving to the hospital, the priorities are the usual: A, B, C, D, E. It is fundamental the correct approach to avoid secondary and irreversible consequences.

When safety is assured, he can be moved to the radiology department to perform the brain and cervical scan ordered by the intensivist.

In the meanwhile, lab results arrived, without major findings; drug panel negative, alcohol negative, coagulation within normal limits.

The Controversial Aspects of Management

In a patient with a GCS of 9, hemodynamically stable, without apparent compromise of the airway (with the Guedel tube to maintain just the patency of the airway), well-oxygenated and well-ventilated, most—not all—intensivists, will not proceed immediately to endotracheal intubation in the absence of signs of vomit. So, while waiting to the results of the CT scan, the patient should be subjected to the secondary and tertiary evaluations, to be sure that in the first exam no lesion has been missed. Admission to an intensive care unit is indicated, due to better conditions for adequate monitoring and treatment in case of deterioration. A neurosurgeon should be contacted.

The neurological status of the patient started to deteriorate, with a GCS of 5 (M3E2V1) and incising pupillary asymmetry. The CT scan became available on the system and show an epidural hematoma. Is this an emergency? Should the neurosurgeon and the operative room be contacted immediately?

The patient was taken to the OR and an epidural hematoma was drained. Transferred to the ICU under sedation, residual effects of neuro-muscular blockers, intubated and ventilated. Neurologically with GCS not evaluable due to sedation, with just a smaller pupillary asymmetry. Six hours later the CT scan was repeated and no complications were seen. Over the next 24 hours sedo-analgesia was slowly withdraw. The patient recovered completely although slowly, without motor deficits and was transferred at 96 h to the neurosurgical ward.

Patients with a Glasgow Coma Scale ≤13 should be rapidly transported as soon as possible to a differentiated hospital with neurosurgery. Also patients with a moderate to severe extra-cranial anatomic injuries and Abbreviated Injury Score ≥3 should also be promptly transferred. Triage is fundamental in pre-hospital assistance to ensure the adequate treatment of the patient. Special care with the airway and ventilation is mandatory, with most authors recommending endo-tracheal intubation when the GCS is <= 8 or if there are signs of vomit; this is main to avoid secondary aspiration and manutention of the patency of the airway, as well as facilitate patient oxygenation.

We know that damage control surgery and/or interventional radiology can be a successful treatment in brain hemorrhage, so it is a preventable death if we do the correct initial evaluation on time. The combination of a correct triage and detailed physical/neurological exam with a CT scan is enough to determine the best approach. Until now we don´t have recommendations that indicate the use of a MRI instead of a CT scan.

In these patients, the priority is to prevent secondary brain injury and avoid morbidity and/or mortality. That type of injury may result from systemic hypotension and hypoxemia and unfortunately there are many cases that present hypoxemia or hypotension.

At present, the defining level of hypotension is unclear. Systolic blood pressure of less than 90 mm Hg, must be rapidly corrected.

The same applies to the definition of hypoxia as apnea cyanosis or a PaO_2 < 60 mm Hg.

The goal for temperature management is normothermia.

The objective for electrolytes is to maintain within normal range. Attention to the sodium level is fundamental. Hyponatremia may worsen cerebral edema. TBI patients may also develop diabetes insipidus, the syndrome of inappropriate antidiuretic hormone, or cerebral salt wasting syndrome. That is why, patients have to be frequently monitored to detect on time serum sodium and osmolality changes.

Glicemia blood levels also have to be monitored because they also influence the outcome in these patients.

Anemia and coagulopathy are common and have to be monitored closely. It is recommended red blood cell transfusion for hemoglobin level <7 g/dl in life-threatening situations. Coagulation assessment can be done using INR or thromboelastography, rotational thromboelastometry, and/or platelet function assays.

ICP monitoring should be done in patients with GCS ≤8 with evidence of structural brain damage. There are some situations when GCS is >8 in which ICP monitoring is indicated, like presence of structural brain damage with high risk for progression. ICP monitoring should also be considered when surgery for extracranial injuries is needed, in case we need to start mechanical ventilation, or in patients that evidence progression of pathology on CT imaging or clinical examination.

ICP monitoring can be done by different methods. Some neurosurgeons will advocate the colocation of an external ventricular drain with ICP monitor because it is both diagnostic and therapeutic. However, most intensivists and neurosurgeons—in the absence of hydrocephaly—will opt for the insertion of an intra-cortical catheter, to measure ICP, temperature and in most cases Pti = 2. Elevated ICP or decreased $PTiO_2$ are independent predictors of poor outcome. Cerebral perfusion pressure (CPP), a parameter derived from ICP (Mean Arterial Pressure – ICP), can also help us to achieve our goal because augmenting CPP may improve perfusion and oxygenation but can also conduct to increased ICP without increased CPP if the patient is out of the auto-regulation window. The identification of ICP elevation implies new imaging and fast intervention. The accepted value for ICP is 20 mm Hg, with a reasonable range of 20–25 mm Hg as an alert for treatment of intracranial hypertension. But these seem to be variable depending on each individual. That is why we need to individualize the limits and the treatments.

If we detect ICP elevation in a CT scan this is an indication for surgical evacuation of a traumatic mass lesion, if existing. When the patient has a large traumatic hematoma a craniotomy is necessary to perform the resection. However, in many patients only contusion focus or diffuse cerebral edema is seen, what prompt to prioritize non-surgical therapy, with decompressive craniotomy reserved for those patients refractory to these measures.

Decompressive Craniectomy (DC) can be performed after evacuation of a hematoma because of the resultant cerebral swelling, and in other situations if it is expected ICP to rise or when there is no indication to surgery. The first line treatment for depressed fractures is surgery to prevent infection, but nonoperative management may be attempted in some cases. Performing a DC is a difficult decision and the potential benefits should be studied as well as the potential complications in each case.

Mannitol or hypotonic saline is effective in reducing ICP, however, there are no guidelines about these approaches. When using these solutions is very important to verify the urinary output specially if it is low. Most authors recommend small bolus of 7.5% saline repeated as needed. But more studies are needed to understand better this management and the influence in prognostic.

Analgesics and sedatives can also be used to control ICP. But it is necessary to balance the side effects. High dose barbiturate therapy or ketamine can also be used as treatment and sometimes they are the only option that results in some patients.

In preventing infections, there are no guidelines that recommend routine catheter exchanges, or use of antibiotics for systemic prophylaxis in intubated patients, as well as early tracheostomy or extubation.

Nutrition is fundamental in these patients that can be a long time in ICU. Nutrition should begin as soon as possible, preferably around 24–48 hours of injury. This is of great importance because early nutritional support is associated with fewer infections and lower mortality. Enteral nutrition must be the first choice.

Pharmacological prophylaxis of deep venous thrombosis and of stress ulcer are commonly used.

When a patient has a mild trauma injury and negative CT, the risk for developing an intracranial lesion is minimal and considering that the patient may be safely discharged. But in every circumstance it is important to inform the patient and the family/care provider about the signals and symptoms that imply a revaluation in the hospital.

REFERENCES

1. Marincowitz C, Lecky FE, Townend W, Borakati A, Fabbri A, Sheldon TA. The risk of deterioration in GCS13-15 patients with traumatic brain injury identified by computed tomography imaging: a systematic review and meta-analysis. J Neurotrauma. 2018;35(5):703–718.

2. Brain Trauma Foundation, American Association of Neurological Surgeons, Congress of Neurological Surgeons. Guidelines for the management of severe traumatic brain injury. J Neurotrauma. 2007;24(suppl 1):S1–S106.
3. Hutchinson P. Randomised evaluation of surgery with craniectomy for uncontrollable elevation of intracranial pressure (RESCUEicp). ISRCTN66202560. DOI: 10.1186/ISRCTN66202560. ISRCTN Registry. 2005. Available at:nhttp://www.isrctn.com/ISRCTN66202560.
4. Cooper DJ, Rosenfeld JV,Murray L, et al. Decompressive craniectomy in diffuse traumatic brain injury. N Engl J Med. 2011;364(16):1493-1502. Erratum appears in N Engl J Med. 2011;365(21):2040.
5. Clifton GL, Valadka A, Zygun D, et al. Very early hypothermia induction in patients with severe brain injury (the National Acute Brain Injury Study: Hypothermia II): a randomised trial. Lancet Neurol. 2011;10(2):131–139.
6. Talving P, Karamanos E, Teixeira PG, et al. Intracranial pressure monitoring in severe head injury: compliance with Brain Trauma Foundation guidelines and effect on outcomes: a prospective study. J Neurosurg. 2013;119(5):1248–1254.
7. Haddad S, Aldawood AS, Alferayan A, Russell NA, Tamim HM, Arabi YM. Relationship between intracranial pressure monitoring and outcomes in severe traumatic brain injury patients. Anaesth Intensive Care. 2011;39(6):1043–1050.
8. Stochetti N, Furlan A, Volta F. Hypoxemia and arterial hypotension at the accident scene in head injury. J Trauma 1996;40:764–767.
9. Pietropaoli JA, Rogers FB, Shackford SR, et al. The deleterious effects of intraoperative hypotension on outcome in patients with severe head injuries. J Trauma 1992;33:403–407.
10. Barry KG, Berman AR. Mannitol infusion. Part III. The acute effect of the intravenous infusion of mannitol on blood and plasma volume. N. Engl. J. Med. 1961;264: 1085–1088.
11. Clifton GL, Miller ER, Choi SC, et al. Lack of effect of induction of hypothermia after acute brain injury. N Engl J Med 2001;344:556–563.
12. Rebuck JA, Murry KR, Rhoney DH, et al. Infection related to intracranial pressure monitors in adults: analysis of risk factors and antibiotic prophylaxis. J Neurol Neurosurg Psy chiatry 2000;69:381–384.
13. Goodman JC, Valadka AB, Gopinath SP, et al. Lactate and excitatory amino acids measured by microdialysis are decreased by pentobarbital coma in head-injured patients. J Neurotrauma 1996;13:549–556.
14. Qiu W, Guo C, Shen H, et al. Effects of unilateral decompressive craniectomy on patients with unilateral acute post-traumatic brain swelling after severe traumatic brain injury. Crit Care. 2009;13(6):R185.
15. 8. Wang X, Dong Y, Qi XQ, Li YM, Huang CG, Hou LJ. Clinical review: efficacy of antimicrobial impregnated catheters in external ventricular drainage - a systematic review and meta-analysis. Crit Care. 2013;17(234):1–11.
16. Lepelletier D, Roquilly A, Demeure dit latte D, et al. Retrospective analysis of the risk factors and pathogens associated with early-onset ventilator-associated pneumonia in surgical-ICU head-trauma patients. J Neurosurg Anesthesiol. 2010;22(1):32–37.
17. Alali AS, Fowler RA, Mainprize TG, et al. Intracranial pressure monitoring in severe traumatic brain injury: results from the American College of Surgeons Trauma Quality Improvement Program. J Neurotrauma. 2013;30(20):1737–1746.
18. Brenner M, Stein DM, Hu PF, Aarabi B, Sheth K, Scalea TM. Traditional systolic blood pressure targets underestimate hypotension-induced secondary brain injury. J Trauma Acute Care Surg. 2012;72(5):1135–1139.
19. Chang JJ, Youn TS, Benson D, et al. Physiologic and functional outcome correlates of brain tissue hypoxia in traumatic brain injury. Crit Care Med. 2009;37(1):283–290.
20. Alderson P, Gadkary C, Signorini DF. Therapeutic hypothermia for head injury. Cochrane Database Syst Rev 2004;4:CD001048.
21. McIntyre LA, Fergusson DA, Hebert PC, et al. Prolonged therapeutic hypothermia after traumatic brain injury in adults: a systematic review. JAMA 2003;289:2992–2999.

22. Stiefel MF, Spiotta A, Gracias VH, et al. Reduced mortality rate in patients with severe traumatic brain injury treated with brain tissue oxygen monitoring. J Neurosurg 2005;103:805–811.
23. Van den Brink WA, van Santbrink H, Steyerberg EW, et al. Brain oxygen tension in severe head injury. Neurosurgery 2000;46:868–878.
24. Kelly PF, Goodale DB, Williams J, et al. Propofol in the treatment of moderate and severe head injury: a randomized, prospective double-blinded pilot trial. J Neurosurg 1999;90:1042–1057.
25. Borzotta AP, Pennings J, Papasadero B, et al. Enteral versus parenteral nutrition after severe closed head injury. J Trauma 1994;37:459–468.
26. Servadei F, Antonelli V, Giuliani G, et al. Evolving lesions in traumatic subarachnoid hemorrhage: prospective study of 110 patients with emphasis on the role of ICP monitor- ing. Acta Neurochir Suppl 2002;81:81–82.

CHAPTER

5

Management of Ventilator-associated Pneumonia

Erika P Plata-Menchaca, Ricard Ferrer

CASE PRESENTATION

A 57-year-old male, with a history of smoking and COPD on domiciliary oxygen therapy, underwent bilateral lung transplantation and was transferred to the ICU for postoperative care. On day 0, he presented left pleural bleeding. On day 7, he underwent percutaneous tracheostomy for prolonged mechanical ventilation due to diaphragmatic palsy and bronchopleural fistula. He had received ceftazidime + amoxicillin-clavulanic acid, nebulized liposomal amphotericin B and ganciclovir for antimicrobial prophylaxis in the perioperative period. The immunosuppressive treatment was tacrolimus + mycophenolate mofetil + corticosteroids. The cultures of the patient and donor were negative. On day 9, a fibrobronchoscopy reported uninterrupted bronchial sutures, and the bronchioalveolar lavage culture was negative. The left intrapleural hematoma was treated by the instillation of intrapleural urokinase. On day 18, he presented purulent tracheal secretions as a sole clinical manifestation, and nebulized colistin was started for empirical treatment of tracheobronchitis. On day 23, a tracheal surveillance culture reported *P. aeruginosa*. On day 30, the patient presented fever, leukocytosis, hemodynamic instability. Respiratory cultures reported *P. aeruginosa* and combined empirical antimicrobial treatment with ceftazidime +amikacin + nebulized colistin was started. Chest X-ray is shown below.

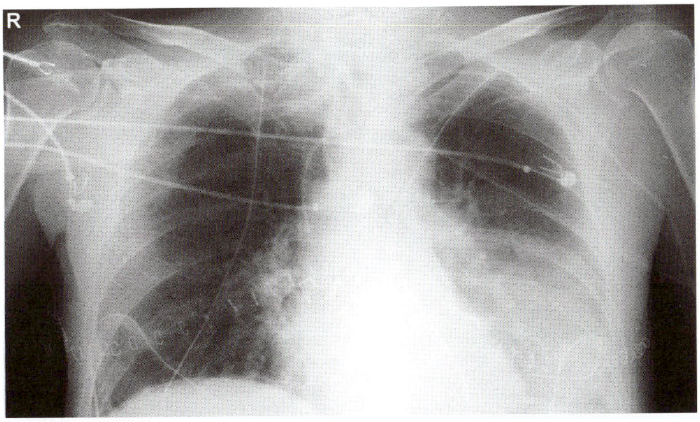

What is the Definition of Ventilator-associated Pneumonia?

Ventilator-associated pneumonia (VAP) is a type of hospital-acquired pneumonia defined as lung infection developing after 48 hours of starting invasive mechanical ventilation.

This condition is considered a severe complication, as it carries a high risk of death among mechanically ventilated critically ill patients. The severity of the disease, infections caused by multidrug-resistant organisms, and wrong empirical therapy in the context of high-drug resistance are associated with the worst prognosis. First, clinicians should differentiate VAP from ventilated hospital-acquired pneumonia, as clinical implications, prognosis, and approach to treatment differ.[1, 2]

VAP is a frequent condition among critically ill patients, also associated with adverse outcomes and high costs.[3,4] In the ICU population, the risk of VAP is approximately 18–40%,[5] and it increases the risk of mortality by 38% at 30 days. However, compared with ICU- or hospital-acquired pneumonia, the risk of 30-day mortality is lower for VAP (82% *vs* 38%).[6] VAP leads to prolonged ICU length of stay and increases the duration of MV.[7] The crude mortality of VAP is reported to range between 24% and 72%. The highest mortality is associated with difficult-to-treat (DTT) *Pseudomonas aeruginosa* infection.[8]

Principles of Empirical and Targeted Management

Diagnosis and definitions: VAP occurs after 48 hours of endotracheal intubation and invasive ventilation. Pneumonia is defined as a new lung infiltrate and clinical evidence that it is of an infectious origin (e.g. the new onset of fever, purulent sputum, leucocytosis) and worsening oxygenation parameters.[9] The 2005 guidelines definition was not modified in the 2016 American guidelines. According to the US Centers for Disease Control and Prevention (CDC), VAP includes the following:[10]

- New or progressive infiltrate, consolidation, or cavitation
- Fever (> 38°C) or leucocytosis (≥12,000 WBC/µL) or leukopenia (<4,000 WBC/µL)
- A positive culture for a pathogenic organism in adequate sputum or bronchoalveolar lavage sample with ≥25 neutrophils in a low-power field and
- Decreasing oxygenation after at least two calendar days of clinical stability (≥2 days of stable or decreasing daily minimum PEEP followed by a rise in daily minimum PEEP of ≥2.5 cm H_2O, sustained for ≥2 days; or ≥2 d of stable or decreasing daily minimum FiO_2 followed by an increase in daily minimum, FiO_2 of ≥0.15 points, sustained for ≥2 days)

These CDC criteria are not useful for diagnosis at the bedside. They were developed to improve surveillance and quality improvement of VAP in hospitals.[11]

Cultures

Cultures of respiratory secretions before initiating therapy are a priority in all cases to narrow broad-spectrum treatments as soon as microbiological information regarding the causative pathogen is obtained. The American guidelines recommend non-invasive samples and semiquantitative cultures rather than invasive samples,[11] and the European Guidelines invasive quantitative samples.[12] Whichever technique is used according to local protocols, the deleterious effects of bronchoscopy on gas exchange in unstable critically ill patients with septic shock or ARDS should be counterbalanced with the benefits of diagnostic techniques.[13] There is a high level of evidence comparing quantitative and qualitative sampling for VAP diagnosis, and there were no differences in mortality or other secondary outcomes.[14, 15] Qualitative diagnostic approaches (e.g. endotracheal aspirates) increases the sensitivity of cultures.[16] However, the overidentification of pathogens carries a risk of overtreatment if the results are not clinically correlated.

Risk factors for VAP: The duration of ventilation is one of the most important risk factors.[17] Therefore, the attributed mortality increases with the time of onset of VAP. Ventilator-associated tracheobronchitis (VAT) is a predisposing condition for VAP.[18] Early-onset VAP has a mortality rate of ~19% and late-onset VAP of ~30%.[13] Reports suggest that secondary infections in critically ill patients with sepsis and high acute severity scores contribute to overall mortality.[19]

- **Patient-related factors:** Different factors are associated with the development of VAP, such as inadequate hand hygiene, inappropriate manipulation of respiratory support devices, severe acute or chronic disease, immunosuppression, prolonged duration of mechanical ventilation, altered level of consciousness, malnutrition, smoking, chronic pulmonary or kidney disease, alcoholism, diabetes mellitus.
- **ICU risk factors:** These include sepsis, ARDS, ECMO, burns, traumatic brain injury, deep or prolonged sedation, thoracic surgery, abdominal surgery, intra-abdominal hypertension, corticosteroids or other immunosuppressive drugs, and overuse of broad-spectrum antimicrobials.[9,11,17,20,21] Hyperoxemia contributes adversely to the development of VAP.[22]

Empirical antimicrobial treatment: VAP is a severe ICU-acquired infection affecting patients' outcomes. Broad-spectrum antibiotics are recommended by international guidelines, with coverage against all likely pathogens. The underlying risk of acquiring multidrug-resistant organisms due to therapy may lead to adverse outcomes and increased mortality. Knowledge of local epidemiology, risk factors for resistance, and microbiological surveillance cultures are tools that improve the prescription of antimicrobials, overall management, and clinical approaches to VAP. The choice of adequate empirical therapy is not a simple process, despite being one of the most important prognostic factors. The use of new-generation rapid and non-invasive diagnostic tests will improve diagnostic approaches and the prescription empiric antibiotic treatment. Their diagnostic accuracy is higher (sensitivity of 89.2%; specificity of 97.1%) than using endotracheal aspirates (sensitivity of 71.8%; specificity of 96.6%). The BioFire FilmArray Blood Culture panel has a specificity of 98.1%, and a negative predictive value is 96.6% for the 1-hour identification of pathogens causing VAP.[23]

Causative pathogens: The most common etiologies are *Enterobacteriaceae spp, P. aeruginosa, S. aureus (methicillin-susceptible-MSSA and methicillin-resistant-MRSA), Acinetobacter spp., Klebsiella spp.*[5] In China, there is a high incidence of MDR pathogens (e.g. carbapenem-resistant *Acinetobacter baumanni*, carbapenem-resistant *Klebsiella pneumoniae* (CKP), carbapenem-resistant *P. aeruginosa*, MRSA, and *S. maltophilia*. The incidence of MDR pathogens is variable among different geographic areas. Knowledge of the local ecology determines the risk of airway colonization and developing VAP.[24]

VAP Caused by Multidrug-resistant Organisms

Local antibiotic resistance is strongly affected by local antibiotic prescription practices.[25] In some areas,[26] there is a high likelihood of receiving inadequate empirical treatment for *P. aeruginosa*, even in patients receiving combination treatment. Microbiological surveillance and local epidemiology aid in decision-making processes.[24] Before choosing empirical antimicrobials in critically ill patients with VAP, different risk factors for MDR organisms should be reviewed.[12]

High prevalence of MDR organisms in the unit or hospital, patients with septic shock, history of recent hospitalization for >5 days, known airway colonization with MDR organisms, and the use of previous or prolonged use of broad-spectrum antibiotics during ICU stay are the most important factors for these infections. Common MDR organisms are difficult-to-treat (DTR): *Pseudomonas aeruginosa*, MRSA, extended-spectrum beta-lactamase-producing enterobacteria (ESBL-E), *Acinetobacter baumannii*, and carbapenemase-producing *Enterobacteriaceae*. Improving antimicrobial stewardship policies help decrease the widespread problem of high MDR prevalence.

In patients colonized by an MDR organism elsewhere, empiric antimicrobial treatment coverage should include the pathogen only if previously described as a potential cause of the suspected infection. Bedside scores can be used to identify cases in which carbapenems could be useful.[27]

Choosing the Most Appropriate Treatment for this Patient

Given that antibiotics are highly valuable drugs, particularly in areas with limited resources, the choice of the best treatment should be rational. Key considerations include prompt de-escalation and awareness of potential side effects and drug interactions.[28, 29]

Rationale

First, establishing the severity of infection, risk factors for resistance, and knowledge of the local ecology in your unit or hospital are needed. Patient's previous colonization and pharmacodynamic/pharmacokinetic properties of antibiotics are other factors to consider. The empirical treatment should consider local ecology, acute severity of the disease, time of diagnosis, previous colonization, comorbidities, the risk for resistance, available drugs, and known efficacy of antibiotics.[30–43]

In sepsis due to VAP,[44] early appropriate broad-spectrum empirical antibiotic treatment should be administered right away.[45] The empirical therapy also targets MDR pathogens colonizing the patient or being prevalent in the unit. Additional diagnostic procedures should not delay the initiation of treatment in severe cases. Novel drugs, such as ceftolozane/tazobactam, ceftazidime/avibactam, and cefiderocol, have been studied for the targeted treatment of MDR: *P. aeruginosa* and ESBL-E. These drugs have acceptable *in vitro* activity and resistance profiles among isolates of MDR pathogens.[30,31]

Cefiderocol is a suitable for DTR: *P. aeruginosa* infections localized outside of the urinary tract. This drug is a synthetic conjugate that binds to iron and facilitates bacterial cell entry using active iron transporters.[46] The cephalosporin moiety of the drug dissociates in the periplasmic space and binds primarily to penicillin-binding protein 3, inhibiting bacterial cell wall synthesis. In previous studies, around 97% of isolates were susceptible to cefiderocol (i.e. MICs ≤4 µg/mL).[47]

A large RCT, the CREDIBLE-CR TRIAL, compared cefiderocol and polymyxin-based therapy for severe infections due to carbapenem-resistant organisms.[48] The trial included 29 DTR: *P. aeruginosa* infections (6 patients had urinary infections, 17 had respiratory tract infections, and 6 had bloodstream infections). Overall mortality was 18% in both arms. Cefiderocol was not inferior to combinations of extended-infusion meropenem, polymyxins, and aminoglycosides. However, cefiderocol was not associated with improved outcomes, as with other β-lactam-β-lactamase inhibitors.[49] Cefiderocol is an alternative when the newer β-lactam-β-lactamase inhibitors cannot be used due to inactivity, intolerance, or unavailability. Tigecycline is not approved for VAP treatment.[50]

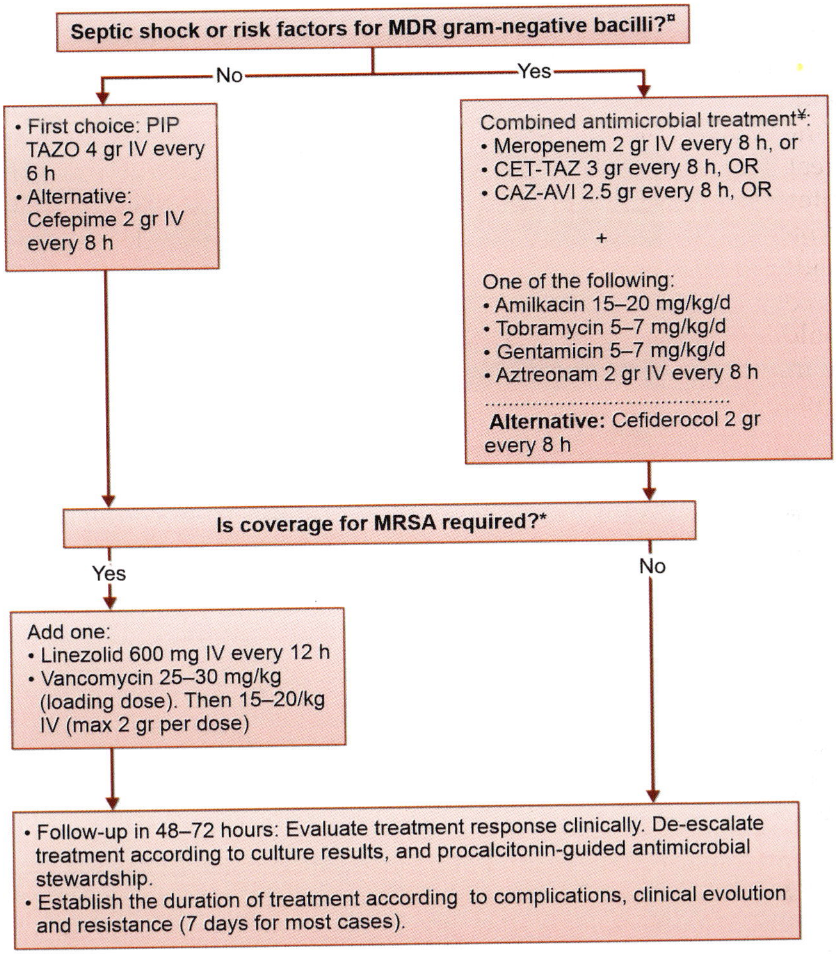

Fig. 5.1: Management algorithm for ventilator-associated pneumonia, according to international guidelines.[35–43] Note that combined treatments with broad-spectrum antimicrobials should be reassessed in 48–72 hours for early de-escalation when indicated. Procalcitonin and other objective tools could aid in decision-making.

MDR denotes multidrug-resistant, CFT-TAZ ceftolozane-tazobactam, CAZ-AVI ceftazidime-avibactam, PIP-TAZO piperacillin-tazobactam, MRSA Methicillin-resistant *S. aureus*.

¥Adjust according to surveillance cultures (previous colonization), local ecology on antimicrobial susceptibility patterns, and rapid diagnostic test if available.

**Risk factors for MRSA*: Age, ARDS, multilobar involvement, colonization by MRSA, recent hospitalization (90 days), nursing home residence, recent exposition to antimicrobials covering gram-positive bacteria.

¤*Risk factors for MDR gram-negative bacilli*: Prior colonization or infection by *P. aeruginosa* or gram-negative bacilli, solid cancer, shock, chronic organ disease, prolonged ICU admission, prior use of carbapenems, prolonged duration of antimicrobial therapy, admission from another healthcare facility, recent exposure to MRSA treatment, systemic illness, invasive devices, high APACHE score.

Duration of Treatment

For most patients, 7-day courses of antimicrobial therapy are recommended by international guidelines to avoid the emergence of resistance. The iDIAPASON trial (*Impact of the Duration of Antibiotics on Clinical Events in Patients With Pseudomonas aeruginosa Ventilator-associated Pneumonia* trial) showed that a short duration versus long duration of treatment of VAP due to *P. aeruginosa* (8 *vs* 15 days) is safe. The authors also demonstrated that shorter treatments did not increase mortality or recurrence rate.[51]

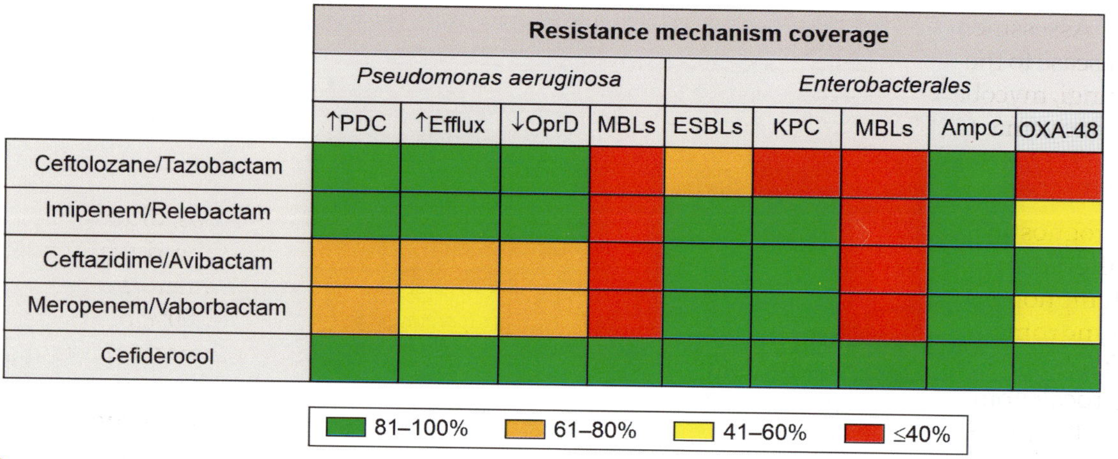

Fig. 5.2: *In vitro* coverage of clinical isolates using CLSI breakpoints based on published studies and MSD internal data

Of note, the optimal duration of therapy for some MDR organisms has not been defined, though antibiotic de-escalation is part of high-quality antimicrobial stewardship (AS) protocols. Considering locally available resources, AS policies could be helpful in decision-making processes and in ensuring appropriate antimicrobial treatments.

The inadvertent use of antimicrobial combinations can induce the emergence of highly resistant strains. Thus, as soon as a causative microorganism is identified in respiratory samples, de-escalation can be done if the clinical status improves 48 to 72 hours after initiating adequate treatment. Procalcitonin-guided treatment could aid in defining duration in some cases, such as initial inadequate treatments, infections due to MDR organisms, or when second-line antibiotics are used.[12] Some experts recommend the use of procalcitonin delta values in combination with objective clinical parameters (e.g. Clinical Pulmonary Infection Score [CPIS], PaO_2/FiO_2, Sequential Organ Failure Assessment [SOFA] score).[52]

Local protocols focusing on the widespread use of antimicrobial stewardship practices considering clinical progression, biomarkers, and microbiological surveillance will aid the early de-escalation of broad-spectrum antibiotics. Novel strategies have been developed to enhance the quality of care of mechanically ventilated patients and VAP prevention.

Clinical Response

Clinical response at day 45 (left), 60 (middle), and 70 (right), respectively.

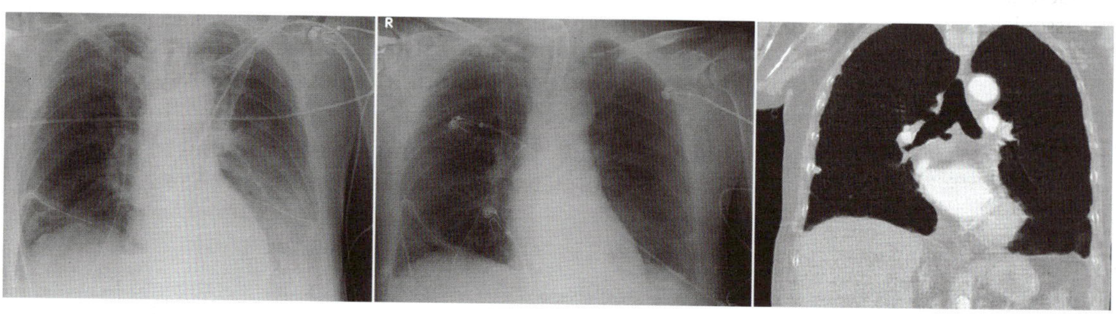

Fig. 5.3: Clinical response at day 45, 60 and 70 respectively

Assessment of clinical non-response should involve the following causes: Attributing the disease to the wrong microorganism, resistant pathogen, additional aetiologies (other bacteria, fungi, mycobacteria, viruses), inadequate antimicrobial therapy, the presence of complications (empyema, *C. difficile* colitis, another focus of infection, drugs, or wrong diagnosis.

Prognosis

Prognostic factors include: Septic shock due to VAP, chronic comorbidities, older age and altered previous functional status, acute severity of disease (multiorgan dysfunction), lymphopenia, malignant neoplasias, the persistence of systemic inflammatory response syndrome and purulent secretions, multilobar infiltrates in more than 50% of the lung fields.[53–55] Clinical scores and antimicrobial management guided by biomarkers, such as procalcitonin, could aid in clinical practice.[52, 56]

The two most important factors determining mortality in cases with VAP are the absence of improved oxygenation during antibiotic treatment and having received adequate antimicrobial treatment.[57] This patient was discharged after 120 days in the ICU.

REFERENCES

1. Saied W, Martin-Loeches I, Timsit JF. What is new in non-ventilated ICU-acquired pneumonia? Intensive Care Med. 2020;46(3):488–91.
2. Zaragoza R, Vidal-Cortés P, Aguilar G, Borges M, Diaz E, Ferrer R, et al. Update of the treatment of nosocomial pneumonia in the ICU. Crit Care. 2020;24(1):383.
3. Warren DK, Shukla SJ, Olsen MA, Kollef MH, Hollenbeak CS, Cox MJ, et al. Outcome and attributable cost of ventilator-associated pneumonia among intensive care unit patients in a suburban medical center. Crit Care Med. 2003;31(5):1312–7.
4. Esperatti M, Ferrer M, Theessen A, Liapikou A, Valencia M, Saucedo LM, et al. Nosocomial pneumonia in the intensive care unit acquired by mechanically ventilated versus nonventilated patients. Am J Respir Crit Care Med. 2010;182(12):1533–9.
5. Koulenti D, Tsigou E, Rello J. Nosocomial pneumonia in 27 ICUs in Europe: perspectives from the EU-VAP/CAP study. Eur J Clin Microbiol Infect Dis. 2017;36(11):1999–2006.
6. Ibn Saied W, Mourvillier B, Cohen Y, Ruckly S, Reignier J, Marcotte G, et al. A Comparison of the Mortality Risk Associated With Ventilator-Acquired Bacterial Pneumonia and Nonventilator ICU-Acquired Bacterial Pneumonia. Crit Care Med. 2019;47(3):345–52.
7. Papazian L, Klompas M, Luyt CE. Ventilator-associated pneumonia in adults: a narrative review. Intensive Care Med. 2020;46(5):888–906.
8. Micek ST, Wunderink RG, Kollef MH, Chen C, Rello J, Chastre J, et al. An international multicenter retrospective study of *Pseudomonas aeruginosa* nosocomial pneumonia: impact of multidrug resistance. Crit Care. 2015;19(1):219.
9. Guidelines for the management of adults with hospital-acquired, ventilator-associated, and healthcare-associated pneumonia. Am J Respir Crit Care Med. 2005;171(4):388–416.
10. Hayashi Y, Morisawa K, Klompas M, Jones M, Bandeshe H, Boots R, et al. Toward improved surveillance: the impact of ventilator-associated complications on length of stay and antibiotic use in patients in intensive care units. Clin Infect Dis. 2013;56(4):471–7.
11. Kalil AC, Metersky ML, Klompas M, Muscedere J, Sweeney DA, Palmer LB, et al. Management of Adults With Hospital-acquired and Ventilator-associated Pneumonia: 2016 Clinical Practice Guidelines by the Infectious Diseases Society of America and the American Thoracic Society. Clin Infect Dis. 2016;63(5):e61–e111.
12. Torres A, Niederman MS, Chastre J, Ewig S, Fernandez-Vandellos P, Hanberger H, et al. International ERS/ESICM/ESCMID/ALAT guidelines for the management of hospital-acquired pneumonia and ventilator-associated pneumonia: Guidelines for the management of hospital-acquired pneumonia (HAP)/ventilator-associated pneumonia (VAP) of the European Respiratory Society (ERS), European Society of Intensive

Care Medicine (ESICM), European Society of Clinical Microbiology and Infectious Diseases (ESCMID) and Asociacion Latinoamericana del Torax (ALAT). Eur Respir J. 2017;50(3).

13. Martin-Loeches I, Rodriguez AH, Torres A. New guidelines for hospital-acquired pneumonia/ventilator-associated pneumonia: USA vs. Europe. Curr Opin Crit Care. 2018;24(5):347–52.
14. Berton DC, Kalil AC, Teixeira PJ. Quantitative versus qualitative cultures of respiratory secretions for clinical outcomes in patients with ventilator-associated pneumonia. Cochrane Database Syst Rev. 2014(10):Cd006482.
15. Canadian Critical Care Trials Group. A randomized trial of diagnostic techniques for ventilator-associated pneumonia. N Engl J Med. 2006;355(25):2619–30.
16. Solé Violán J, Fernández JA, Benítez AB, Cardeñosa Cendrero JA, Rodríguez de Castro F. Impact of quantitative invasive diagnostic techniques in the management and outcome of mechanically ventilated patients with suspected pneumonia. Crit Care Med. 2000;28(8):2737–41.
17. Wu D, Wu C, Zhang S, Zhong Y. Risk Factors of Ventilator-Associated Pneumonia in Critically Ill Patients. Front Pharmacol. 2019;10:482.
18. Martin-Loeches I, Povoa P, Rodríguez A, Curcio D, Suarez D, Mira JP, et al. Incidence and prognosis of ventilator-associated tracheobronchitis (TAVeM): a multicentre, prospective, observational study. Lancet Respir Med. 2015;3(11):859–68.
19. van Vught LA, Klein Klouwenberg PM, Spitoni C, Scicluna BP, Wiewel MA, Horn J, et al. Incidence, Risk Factors, and Attributable Mortality of Secondary Infections in the Intensive Care Unit After Admission for Sepsis. Jama. 2016;315(14):1469–79.
20. Forel JM, Voillet F, Pulina D, Gacouin A, Perrin G, Barrau K, et al. Ventilator-associated pneumonia and ICU mortality in severe ARDS patients ventilated according to a lung-protective strategy. Crit Care. 2012;16(2):R65.
21. Li Y, Liu C, Xiao W, Song T, Wang S. Incidence, Risk Factors, and Outcomes of Ventilator-Associated Pneumonia in Traumatic Brain Injury: A Meta-analysis. Neurocrit Care. 2020;32(1):272–85.
22. Jaffal K, Six S, Zerimech F, Nseir S. Relationship between hyperoxemia and ventilator associated pneumonia. Ann Transl Med. 2017;5(22):453.
23. Pulido MR, Moreno-Martínez P, González-Galán V, Fernández Cuenca F, Pascual Á, Garnacho-Montero J, et al. Application of BioFire FilmArray Blood Culture Identification panel for rapid identification of the causative agents of ventilator-associated pneumonia. Clin Microbiol Infect. 2018;24(11):1213.e1–.e4.
24. Bonten MJ, Weinstein RA. The role of colonization in the pathogenesis of nosocomial infections. Infect Control Hosp Epidemiol. 1996;17(3):193–200.
25. Beardsley JR, Williamson JC, Johnson JW, Ohl CA, Karchmer TB, Bowton DL. Using local microbiologic data to develop institution-specific guidelines for the treatment of hospital-acquired pneumonia. Chest. 2006;130(3):787–93.
26. ENVIN - HELICS [Internet]. [cited 2020 Nov 3]. Available from: http://hws.vhebron.net/envin-helics/https://hws.vhebron.net/envin-helics/Help/Informe%20ENVIN-UCI%202019.pdf.
27. Teysseyre L, Ferdynus C, Miltgen G, Lair T, Aujoulat T, Lugagne N, et al. Derivation and validation of a simple score to predict the presence of bacteria requiring carbapenem treatment in ICU-acquired bloodstream infection and pneumonia: CarbaSCORE. Antimicrob Resist Infect Control. 2019;8:78.
28. Tabah A, Bassetti M, Kollef MH, Zahar JR, Paiva JA, Timsit JF, et al. Antimicrobial de-escalation in critically ill patients: a position statement from a task force of the European Society of Intensive Care Medicine (ESICM) and European Society of Clinical Microbiology and Infectious Diseases (ESCMID) Critically Ill Patients Study Group (ESGCIP). Intensive Care Med. 2020;46(2):245–65.
29. Ruiz J, Ramirez P, Gordon M, Villarreal E, Frasquet J, Poveda-Andres JL, et al. Antimicrobial stewardship programme in critical care medicine: A prospective interventional study. Med Intensiva. 2018;42(5):266–73.
30. Bassetti M, Righi E, Vena A, Graziano E, Russo A, Peghin M. Risk stratification and treatment of ICU-acquired pneumonia caused by multidrug- resistant/extensively drug-resistant/pandrug-resistant bacteria. Curr Opin Crit Care. 2018;24(5):385–93.
31. Montravers P, Bassetti M. The ideal patient profile for new beta-lactam/beta-lactamase inhibitors. Curr Opin Infect Dis. 2018;31(6):587–93.
32. Bassetti M, Vena A, Russo A, Croxatto A, Calandra T, Guery B. Rational approach in the management of *Pseudomonas aeruginosa* infections. Curr Opin Infect Dis. 2018;31(6):578–86.

33. Mensa J, Barberán J, Soriano A, Llinares P, Marco F, Cantón R, et al. Antibiotic selection in the treatment of acute invasive infections by *Pseudomonas aeruginosa*: Guidelines by the Spanish Society of Chemotherapy. Rev Esp Quimioter. 2018;31(1):78–100.
34. Bassetti M, Righi E, Carnelutti A, Graziano E, Russo A. Multidrug-resistant Klebsiella pneumoniae: challenges for treatment, prevention and infection control. Expert Rev Anti Infect Ther. 2018;16(10):749–61.
35. Freire AT, Melnyk V, Kim MJ, Datsenko O, Dzyublik O, Glumcher F, et al. Comparison of tigecycline with imipenem/cilastatin for the treatment of hospital-acquired pneumonia. Diagn Microbiol Infect Dis. 2010;68(2):140–51.
36. Rubinstein E, Lalani T, Corey GR, Kanafani ZA, Nannini EC, Rocha MG, et al. Telavancin versus vancomycin for hospital-acquired pneumonia due to gram-positive pathogens. Clin Infect Dis. 2011;52(1):31–40.
37. Kollef MH, Chastre J, Clavel M, Restrepo MI, Michiels B, Kaniga K, et al. A randomized trial of 7-day doripenem versus 10-day imipenem-cilastatin for ventilator-associated pneumonia. Crit Care. 2012;16(6):R218.
38. Wunderink RG, Niederman MS, Kollef MH, Shorr AF, Kunkel MJ, Baruch A, et al. Linezolid in methicillin-resistant *Staphylococcus aureus* nosocomial pneumonia: a randomized, controlled study. Clin Infect Dis. 2012;54(5):621–9.
39. Ramirez J, Dartois N, Gandjini H, Yan JL, Korth-Bradley J, McGovern PC. Randomized phase 2 trial to evaluate the clinical efficacy of two high-dosage tigecycline regimens versus imipenem-cilastatin for treatment of hospital-acquired pneumonia. Antimicrob Agents Chemother. 2013;57(4):1756–62.
40. Awad SS, Rodriguez AH, Chuang YC, Marjanek Z, Pareigis AJ, Reis G, et al. A phase 3 randomized double-blind comparison of ceftobiprole medocaril versus ceftazidime plus linezolid for the treatment of hospital-acquired pneumonia. Clin Infect Dis. 2014;59(1):51–61.
41. Torres A, Zhong N, Pachl J, Timsit JF, Kollef M, Chen Z, et al. Ceftazidime-avibactam versus meropenem in nosocomial pneumonia, including ventilator-associated pneumonia (REPROVE): a randomised, double-blind, phase 3 non-inferiority trial. Lancet Infect Dis. 2018;18(3):285–95.
42. Cisneros JM, Rosso-Fernández CM, Roca-Oporto C, De Pascale G, Jiménez-Jorge S, Fernández-Hinojosa E, et al. Colistin versus meropenem in the empirical treatment of ventilator-associated pneumonia (Magic Bullet study): an investigator-driven, open-label, randomized, noninferiority controlled trial. Crit Care. 2019;23(1):383.
43. Kollef MH, Nováček M, Kivistik Ü, Réa-Neto Á, Shime N, Martin-Loeches I, et al. Ceftolozane-tazobactam versus meropenem for treatment of nosocomial pneumonia (ASPECT-NP): a randomised, controlled, double-blind, phase 3, non-inferiority trial. Lancet Infect Dis. 2019;19(12):1299–311.
44. Singer M, Deutschman CS, Seymour CW, Shankar-Hari M, Annane D, Bauer M, et al. The Third International Consensus Definitions for Sepsis and Septic Shock (Sepsis-3). Jama. 2016;315(8):801–10.
45. Rhodes A, Evans LE, Alhazzani W, Levy MM, Antonelli M, Ferrer R, et al. Surviving Sepsis Campaign: International Guidelines for Management of Sepsis and Septic Shock: 2016. Intensive Care Med. 2017;43(3):304–77.
46. McCreary EK, Heil EL, Tamma PD. New Perspectives on Antimicrobial Agents: Cefiderocol. Antimicrob Agents Chemother. 2021;65(8):e0217120.
47. Tamma PD, Aitken SL, Bonomo RA, Mathers AJ, van Duin D, Clancy CJ. Infectious Diseases Society of America Antimicrobial-Resistant Treatment Guidance: Gram-Negative Bacterial Infections. Infectious Diseases Society of America 2022; Version 1.1. Available at https://www.idsociety.org/practice-guideline/amr-guidance/. Accessed 26/11/2022.
48. Bassetti M, Echols R, Matsunaga Y, Ariyasu M, Doi Y, Ferrer R, et al. Efficacy and safety of cefiderocol or best available therapy for the treatment of serious infections caused by carbapenem-resistant Gram-negative bacteria (CREDIBLE-CR): a randomised, open-label, multicentre, pathogen-focused, descriptive, phase 3 trial. Lancet Infect Dis. 2020.
49. Pogue JM, Kaye KS, Veve MP, Patel TS, Gerlach AT, Davis SL, et al. Ceftolozane/Tazobactam vs Polymyxin or Aminoglycoside-based Regimens for the Treatment of Drug-resistant *Pseudomonas aeruginosa*. Clin Infect Dis. 2020;71(2):304–10.
50. FDA Drug Safety Communication: Increased risk of death with Tygacil (tigecycline) compared to other antibiotics used to treat similar infections. Accessed November 10, 2020. https://www.fda.gov/drugs/drug-

safety-and-availability/fda-drug-safety-communication-increased-risk-death-tygacil-tigecycline-compared-other-antibiotics.

51. Bouglé A, Foucrier A, Dupont H, Montravers P, Ouattara A, Kalfon P, et al. Impact of the duration of antibiotics on clinical events in patients with *Pseudomonas aeruginosa* ventilator-associated pneumonia: study protocol for a randomized controlled study. Trials. 2017;18(1):37.
52. Torres A, Artigas A, Ferrer R. Biomarkers in the ICU: less is more? No. Intensive Care Med. 2020:1–4.
53. Ranzani OT, Ferrer M, Esperatti M, Giunta V, Bassi GL, Carvalho CR, et al. Association between systemic corticosteroids and outcomes of intensive care unit-acquired pneumonia. Crit Care Med. 2012;40(9):2552–61.
54. Ranzani OT, Prina E, Torres A. Nosocomial pneumonia in the intensive care unit: how should treatment failure be predicted? Rev Bras Ter Intensiva. 2014;26(3):208–11.
55. Ceccato A, Panagiotarakou M, Ranzani OT, Martin-Fernandez M, Almansa-Mora R, Gabarrus A, et al. Lymphocytopenia as a Predictor of Mortality in Patients with ICU-Acquired Pneumonia. J Clin Med. 2019;8(6).
56. Póvoa P, Martin-Loeches I, Ramirez P, Bos LD, Esperatti M, Silvestre J, et al. Biomarkers kinetics in the assessment of ventilator-associated pneumonia response to antibiotics - results from the BioVAP study. J Crit Care. 2017;41:91–7.
57. Esperatti M, Ferrer M, Giunta V, Ranzani OT, Saucedo LM, Li Bassi G, et al. Validation of predictors of adverse outcomes in hospital-acquired pneumonia in the ICU. Crit Care Med. 2013;41(9):2151–61.

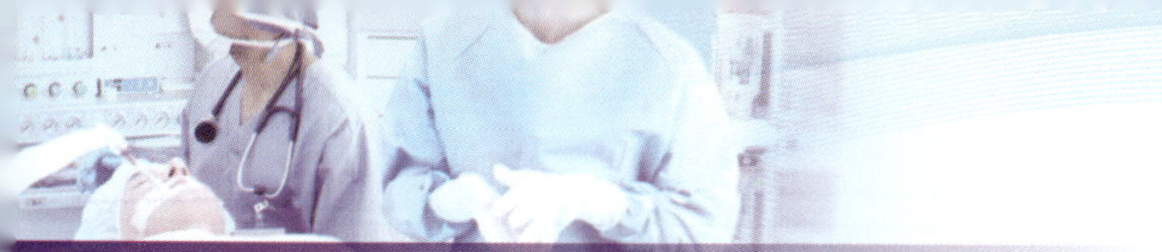

CHAPTER

6

Shock: Diagnosis and Management

Ahsina Jahan Lopa, Dipanjan Chatterjee, Ahsan Ahmed

INTRODUCTION

Shock is a condition characterized by acute circulatory failure leading to inadequate tissue perfusion and resultant widespread hypoxia at cellular level leading to end-organ dysfunction.[1,2] Shock is a medical emergency with high mortality rate which needs prompt management.[3] Shock is usually associated with hypotension (systolic blood pressure <90 mmHg) though normal blood pressure does not always ensure adequate global tissue perfusion.[4]

STAGES OF SHOCK

In response to tissue hypoperfusion, initially there is activation of adrenergic autonomic nervous system which results in venoconstriction, followed by vasoconstriction in all non-essential arterial beds.[2] Cardiac contractility is maximized in an attempt to optimize cardiac output and maintain adequate perfusion pressure to the coronary arteries and brain.[2] Further compensatory mechanisms are activated in the kidney. The renin-angiotensin-aldosterone axis is activated to maintain adequate preload by retention of salt and water. But eventually these compensatory mechanisms fail and patient becomes hypotensive.

There are 4 stages of shock: (i) The primary stage in which the tissues are hypoperfused and anaerobic metabolism is activated and there is accumulation of lactic acid; (ii) Compensated stage in which certain levels of tissue perfusion in vital organs are maintained with compensatory mechanisms; (iii) Progressive stage in which compensatory mechanisms even fail to maintain adequate tissue perfusion of the vital organs and (iv) Irreversible stage in which restoration of perfusion will be ineffective due to permanent loss of tissue and cell.[5]

Mechanisms of Shock

Pathophysiologic mechanisms that can give rise to shock may be one of the following four categories:[1,3]

1. Hypovolemic shock
2. Cardiogenic shock
3. Distributive shock
4. Obstructive shock.

Variable degrees of overlapping may be present in a particular clinical scenario; for example, a patient presenting with cardiogenic shock may have secondary sepsis. In septic shock again, there may be impaired myocardial contractility due to inflammatory toxin and tissue hypoxia induced myocardial dysfunction.

Hypovolemic Shock

Hypovolemic shock occurs due to intravascular volume depletion which results in decreased preload, decreased stroke volume and decreased cardiac output with compensatory increase in systemic vascular resistance.[6,7]

Causes of hypovolemic shock

- Hemorrhagic shock (due to acute blood loss from trauma, variceal bleeding, aortic aneurysm rupture, etc.)
- Severe intravascular fluid depletion due to gastrointestinal loss (diarrhea, vomiting), loss through kidney (due to large diuresis like diabetes insipidus) or third space loss from pancreatitis, burns, etc.

Cardiogenic Shock

It occurs due to inability of cardiac pump to generate blood flow that is adequate enough to maintain tissue oxygenation. There is reduced cardiac output due to decreased cardiac contractility leading to reduced stroke volume with compensated increase in preload and systemic vascular resistance.

Causes of cardiogenic shock

1. Acute myocardial infarction or its complications like papillary muscle rupture or free ventricular wall rupture
2. Cardiomyopathy—dilated, restrictive or hypertrophic
3. Myocarditis
4. Severe stenotic or regurgitant valvular disease
5. Orthotopic transplant rejection
6. Cardiac trauma or tamponade
7. Abnormal heart rates and rythms (brady and tachyarrhythmias).

Distributive Shock

Distributive shock results from severe systemic vasodilatation leading to significant reduction in venous return characterized by reduced preload and low systemic vascular resistance. Because of decreased venous return, resulting from increased venous capacitance, cardiac output may decrease.[8]

Causes of distributive shock

- Sepsis
- Anaphylaxis
- Neurogenic shock
- Adrenal crisis, thyroid storm.

Almost 40% of distributive shock of septic origin has transient cardiomyopathy.[9] These patients have poor prognosis and may present with features of distributive shock along with septic shock.[10]

Obstructive Shock

Conditions such as cardiac tamponade, tension pneumothorax, intra-abdominal hypertension can cause obstructive shock.[11,12] Massive pulmonary embolism is another condition, where effective preload of left ventricle is reduced as there is obstruction of the outflow pathway from right ventricle.[13] In obstructive shock, there is decreased preload, increased systemic vascular resistance and decreased cardiac output like hypovolemic shock.

Causes of obstructive shock

- Tension pneumothorax
- Cardiac tamponade
- Abdominal compartment syndrome
- Pulmonary embolism.

Clinical Features

Presence of more than one of the following clinical features, indicate that the patient is in shock:[14]

- Altered mental status: Anxiety, agitation, drowsiness
- Tachycardia, with shock index (heart rate/systolic blood pressure) >0.8. The change in heart rate may be non-specific as, the base line heart rate may be normal in young patients or fit older patients or patients with certain medications (beta-blockers).[15]
- Bradycardia, heart rate <45/min.
- Tachypnoea (respiratory rate >22/min)
- Hypotension: Systolic BP <90 mmHg; low diastolic blood pressure suggests arterial vasodilation seen in conditions of distributive shock; whereas, a narrow pulse pressure <35 mmHg in indicative of vasoconstrictive conditions such as cardiogenic shock, hypovolemic shock or obstructive shock.[16] Older patients or patients with severe atherosclerosis may have normal systolic blood pressure.[17]
- Acute oliguria
- Mottled skin, cool extremities
- Arterial base deficit of more than -5 mEq/L or lactate >4 mmol/L
- Low mixed venous saturation.

CASE SCENARIO 1

A 70-year-old male patient presented in emergency with altered sensorium for last 1 day. He is known patient of coronary artery disease and had undergone coronary artery bypass grafting (CABG) 1 month back. He has history of cough and cold for last 4–5 days. Post-CABG he needed prolong inotropic supports and his previous echo showed poor LV function. On examination: BP: 90/50 mmHg, Heart rate: 130/min, regular rhythm (ECG: sinus), SpO_2: 92% in room air. Chest B/L fine creps present, respiratory rate: 35/min. ABG: Mixed respiratory and metabolic acidosis. Extremities were cold and clammy. ECG showed ST elevation in anterior leads. Echo screening showed gross biventricular dysfunction, mitral regurgitation.

The above case scenario is an example of cardiogenic shock. The management of a patient in cardiogenic shock includes the following:

Assessment

- Basic monitoring such as continuous ECG, automated non-invasive blood pressure monitoring, oxygen saturation monitoring should be established quickly.[1] Intravenous access is to be set up preferably with at least two large bore peripheral lines.[1] An arterial line is to be secured in unstable patients.
- Enquire about: Chest pain and cardiac history: Consider previous ECG, echocardiography, cardiac shadow in chest radiographs. Anterior classic anginal chest pain will certainly indicate towards cardiogenic shock etiologies; shearing chest pain and back pain with background of hypertension should also be evaluated for aortic dissection.

- Presence of peripheral edema, raised jugular venous pressure, bilateral fine creps on auscultation, positive hepato-jugular reflex, are commonly associated with heart failure leading to cardiogenic shock.[18] Arrhythmias present with irregular rhythm in pulses.

Investigations

- **ECG:** It may show evidence of myocardial infarction, ischemia, arrhythmias. Continuous ECG monitoring is indicated in such conditions. ECG will also help to detect right heart strain pattern in pulmonary embolism, signs of electrolyte abnormalities.[18,19,20]
- **Echocardiography:** Early echocardiography helps to determine the cause of cardiogenic shock. Regional wall motion abnormality is present early in myocardial infarction. Echo helps to detect causes like ruptured ventricular septum, free left ventricular wall rupture, cardiac tamponade, papillary muscle rupture leading to acute severe mitral regurgitation.[21]
- **CXR:** Pulmonary edema, bilateral perihilar opacity, the presence of Kerley B lines, cardiomegaly, and bilateral pleural effusions are usually present in the setting of heart failure.
- **Cardiac enzymes:** There are many biochemical markers to indicate myocardial damage which include: Troponin I and troponin T, LDH, myoglobin, creatine kinase (CK), etc. However, troponin I and troponin T are most widely used in this purpose.
- **Lactate:** Any rise in lactate of >2 mmol/L is a marker of shock.[22,23] Serial lactate is to be examined. Serum lactate levels especially lactate clearance has been found to have prognostic value in patients with septic shock, trauma and cardiac arrest[1]
- **Brain natriuretic peptide (BNP)** is often used as an indicator of acute congestive heart failure (CHF) and as a good prognostic marker.[1]
- **Coronary angiography:** Patients with cardiogenic shock often found to have multivessel coronary artery disease (CAD) in coronary angiography. On coronary angiography ≈15% patients are found to have significant left main lesions and >50% have triple-vessel disease.[24] 80% of cardiogenic shock results from acute myocardial infarction (AMI), leading to ventricular dysfunction. Among the other causes, ventricular septal (4%) or free wall rupture (2%), and acute severe mitral regurgitation (7%) are less frequent than AMI.[25]

Treatment

- Patients, having altered mental status or very unstable hemodynamics need intubation and ventilatory support, as these interventions protect airways and reduce the work of breathing and thus reduces oxygen demand in the setting of shock-induced cellular hypoxia.[1] While intubating, care should be given to choose appropriate medications as inducing agents, appropriate dosage, to avoid further hypotension.
- Non-invasive ventilation may be considered in patients who are having left heart failure with severe dyspnoea in emergency situation or as an adjunct to medical therapy when the patient has failed to respond to improve hypoxaemia and cardiac output.[23,26]
- **Fluid therapy:** Assessment of intravascular volume status may be difficult to perform clinically as signs of hypovolemia such as tachycardia, hypotension, cold clammy extremities are non-specific.[1] In this regard goal directed echocardiography is a bed side tool which should be used to clarify or confirm the etiology and fluid responsiveness.[22,23] A pulmonary artery catheter, helps in continuous hemodynamic monitoring, including precise measurements of fluid states, central venous oxygen saturation and response to therapy, by measuring cardiac index.[27]

- **Vasoactive agents:** Shock with inadequate cardiac function needs inotropic support to maintain cardiac output once the preload is optimized.[28] Vasopressors agents should be titrated to maintain a mean arterial pressure of >65 mm Hg. However, in severely dysfunctional heart, increase in afterload due to vasopressor is likely to be counter-productive. Though there is no definitive concensus regarding choice of vasopressor in cardiogenic shock. Norepinephrine is usually used as first line vasopressor as it is associated with fewer incidence of arrhythmias compared to other vasopressors.[29] Patients with relatively stable blood pressure but signs of severe hypoperfusion, may benefit by the use of inodilators; dobutamine, levosimendan, milrinone. However, these agents may cause hypotension in presence of severe left ventricular dysfunction. Adrenaline infusion has been used in cardiogenic shock patients with severe unstable hemodynamics and ventricular dysfunction. However, the use of adrenaline may be associated with increase in lactate concentration and increased risk of arrhythmias.
- **Mechanical circulatory supports:** Patients, who are not stable with inotropes, need mechanical circulatory supports such as IABP (intra-aortic balloon counterpulsation). ECMO (extra-corporeal membrane oxygenation) or LVAD (left ventricular assist devices).
- **IABP:** IABP is to be considered in patients with cardiogenic shock who are not stable on inotropes and have no contraindications. It acts as a bridge to revascularization as well as recovery after revascularization in patients with myocardial stunning. It augments central aortic pressure and vital organ perfusion including coronary blood flow, and reduces afterload and myocardial oxygen demand.[30]
- **ECMO:** Veno-arterial ECMO has been used to rescue patients with refractory cardiogenic shock arising from various pathology including myocardial infarction, post-cardiac surgery ventricular dysfunction, intractable arrhythmias, intoxications, etc.[31,32] ECMO is an advanced life-saving measure, which can be used as bridge to definitive therapy such as revascularization, transplant or as a bridge to ventricular assist devices.
- **LVAD:** There are multiple ventricular assist devices which are used in refractory cardiogenic shock patients when medical therapy or IABP are ineffective. The LVAD works by increasing the collateral blood flow by maintaining the cardiac output and aortic pressure.[33,34,35] The basic mechanism is pumping the blood from left ventricle to aorta.
- Definitive management of causes:
  - All patients presented with symptoms of acute coronary syndrome should get a coronary angiography done and treated accordingly. Arrhythmias are to be corrected by medical therapy, electrical cardio-version or temporary pacing as per indications.

CASE SCENARIO 2

A patient presenting to emergency department in altered mental state with history of multiple episodes of vomiting, and diarrhoea. On examination his pulse is 130/min, regular rhythm, BP: 100/50 mmHg, SpO_2: 96% in room air. ECG sinus tachycardia. ABG: High anion gap metabolic acidosis, with raised lactate. Extremities cold, peripheral pulse feeble, tongue dry.

CASE SCENARIO 3

A 30-year-old male patient coming in emergency with road traffic accident, with minor external injuries but inability to move his right limb which is extremely swollen, tender to touch at the thigh area. He is drowsy, having heart rate of 125/min, BP: 80/50 mmHg. Cold extremities and feeble peripheral pulse. ABG shows Hb of 7.5 gm/dl, lactate 4 mmol/L, metabolic acidosis. Bed side X-ray lower limb showed fracture neck femur.

Both these cases of shock are arising from hypovolemia. They need fluid resuscitation; first patient with crystalloid and the second one preferentially with packed RBCs.

Hypovolemic Shock

Initial stabilization and assessment: Initial stabilization by maintaining airway, if needed ventilation, intravenous access and principles of fluid therapy are same as in any other shock state. While assessing the patient, look for:

- Recent procedures or trauma: Patients with hypovolemic shock may present with obvious history of trauma or loss of body fluids.
- Fever: May suggest underlying infection.
- Abdominal pain: May indicate ruptured aneurysm (loin pain), sepsis with pelvic or abdominal source causing distributive shock, ruptured ectopic pregnancy or twisted ovarian cyst, diabetic ketoacidosis may present as abdominal pain and manifest as hypovolemic shock (hemorrhagic shock).[22]
- History of diarrhoea and vomiting, block stool, etc.
- There will be narrow pulse pressure, mottled skin, cold, clammy extremities.[16,17]

Diagnostic Tools

Based on the patient's presentation, initial laboratory investigations include:

- **Complete blood count:** Haemoglobin level may give some idea regarding the underlying cause such as haemorrhage. Although, results are non-specific and may be normal in the early stages.[36]
- **Urea, creatinine:** Disproportionately raised urea may be present in hypovolemic shock such as in hemorrhage, dehydration.[37]
- **Extended electrolytes (including Ca/Mg/Phos):** Hyperkalaemia is commonly present in trauma patients, in shock which has progressed to acute kidney injury, in diabetic ketoacidosis. Hypovolemic shock resulting from vomiting and diarrhoea will cause hypokalemia.[37]
- **Coagulation studies:** Coagulation parameters may be deranged trauma patients. It is also rational to check the baseline coagulation parameters as these patients commonly need invasive lines.[38]
- **Lactate:** To be checked like in any other shock state.
- **Chest X-ray:** It may reveal the underlying cause of shock in trauma patients.
- Point of care ultrasonography: USG provides important information such as IVC compressibility suggests fluid requirement, signs of peritoneal collection (bleeding), ruptured ectopic pregnancy.
- **CT scan:** To be used in patients with major trauma, suspected ruptured aortic aneurysm, or intra-abdominal collection, pulmonary embolism.
- Pregnancy test in any patient of reproductive age, presented in shock state of unknown origin.

Treatment

- Intubation and ventilatory support are indicated as with other causes of shock.
- Two large bore peripheral venous cannulas should be placed for bolus crystalloids administration immediately. Mechanical transfusion device can be used in this regard for rapid fluid infusion. To give a fluid challenge, crystalloid solutions, normal saline or

Hartmann's solution is used. To assess fluid responsiveness, there are some static indicators such as: Heart rate, blood pressure, capillary refill time, and central venous pressure. Central venous pressure has been used for a long time as a surrogate to determine fluid requirement as it corroborates with the right ventricular preload. However, in the critical patients, due to complex nature of the underlying pathology, central venous pressure may not correlate with right ventricular end diastolic volume.[1,39,40] Among the dynamic indicators, passive leg rising test is a rapid, non-invasive technique that has been found to be a highly sensitive and specific in detecting fluid responsiveness.[39] Echo cardiography used to assess IVC compressibility, end-diastolic volume, and features such as, non-dilated right heart chambers, a non-displaced intra-ventricular septum, absence of right and left ventricular systolic failure suggest fluid requirement.[41] Pulse pressure variability (measured by specialized haemodynamic monitors) of >13% is another marker of volume responsiveness in mechanically ventilated patients. SVV of more than 12% accurately predicts fluid responsiveness.

- Hypovolemic patients, sustaining trauma and hemorrhage, should be given crystalloids with caution as aggressive fluid resuscitation with crystalloids has been found to be associated with abdominal compartment syndrome, acute respiratory distress syndrome, nosocomial infections and increased number of death.[1,42,43,44]
- Patients with hemorrhagic shock should be managed with blood products.[1] Studies have shown that transfusion of only RBCs and crystalloids in trauma patients, may result in coagulopathy by creating low plasma: RBC ratio. This has been found to be associated with increased incidence of mortality.[45]
- Massive transfusion protocol varies from institution, but the idea is to mimic fresh whole blood transfusion in trauma patients, by transfusing: Packed RBCs, platelets, and fresh frozen plasma. The ratio of these three products also varies among the institutions; from 1:1:1 to lower ratios of platelets.[46]
- Cryoprecipitate, fibrinogen concentrate, and recombinant factor VIIIa have been used with mixed results.
- Potential complications of massive transfusion include metabolic alkalosis, hypocalcemia, hypothermia, and hyperkalemia. These should be managed accordingly.
- Early control of bleeding is a must in hemorrhagic shock.
- Hypovolemic shock due to other reasons such as: Diabetic ketoacidosis, pancreatitis, burns etc, needs specific treatment along with measures to stabilize the hemodynamics.

CASE SCENARIO 4

A 34-year-old patient underwent double valve replacement surgery and was shifted to cardio-thoracic ICU in stable condition. Three hours post-operatively, patient started to have low blood pressure. Initially it responded to IV fluid, but there was progressive rise in CVP. Collection in the mediastinal drain was insignificant. Transesophageal echocardiography was done and collection around the heart particularly at the right ventricular outflow tract was seen. Patient was having cardiac tamponade and was immediately taken for re-exploration.

CASE SCENARIO 5

An 80-year-old male patient presented in the emergency with respiratory distress of sudden onset. On examination, he had diminished breath sounds in the right chest. Heart rate was 125/min, BP: 98/50 mmHg. Patient has long history of smoking and he was on inhaler (seroflow). Chest X-ray showed pneumothorax on the right side.

Above case scenarios are examples of obstructive shock. The management of obstructive shock is principally to clear the obstruction which is causing reduction in cardiac preload. Because the mechanism is hypovolemia due to reduced preload, initial stabilization is like that of hypovolemic shock in most clinical conditions. Pulmonary embolism, on the other hand, may present like cardiogenic shock, and there may be the need of rescue veno-arterial ECMO in the setting of severe cardiac dysfunction in spite of steep inotropic support.

There may be:
- Muffled or quiet heart sounds: Feature of cardiac tamponade
- Absent breath sounds: May be due to tension pneumothorax
- History of venous thromboembolic disease.

Diagnosis can be made by:
- Chest X-ray: To detect tension pneumothorax
- ECG: There may be right heart strain pattern in pulmonary embolism
- Echocardiography: Detects any pericardial collection, right ventricular strain may be sign of pulmonary embolism.
- CT scan: Helps to detect pulmonary embolism, abdominal compartment syndrome.

Definitive treatments are:
- Pneumothorax: Intercostal drain insertion.
- Cardiac tamponade: Paracentesis or re-exploration in post-surgical case.
- Pulmonary embolism is treated by: Thrombolysis or pulmonary embolectomy.

CASE SCENARIO 6

A 50-year-old female patient, on 5th postoperative day following CABG surgery, had signs of confusion, with little restlessness. Her ABG showed: Normal blood gases, with mild rise in base excess and lactate. She was already on noradrenaline support, but had blood pressure of 98/40 mmHg. Previously she had diastolic pressure of persistently more than 60 mmHg. The area under the arterial trace curve was low. There was rise in her TLC from 8 k to 14 k. Her heart rate was 110/min. Face flushed, extremities warm, with palpable bounding pulses. Over next 4 hrs, her hemodynamics worsened, patient became more drowsy. Lab investigations were sent which showed CRP >300, ProCal >4.

This case scenario is suggestive of septic shock (type of distributive shock).

Assessing Septic Shock

- qSOFA score: It is a simple, rapidly calculated scoring system to assess the organ dysfunction and poor outcome. Parameters include:
  - Respiratory rate at least 22 breaths/minute
  - Systolic blood pressure 100 mm Hg or lower
  - Altered mental status (Glasgow Coma Scale score <15).

  Patients having a qSOFA score of 2 or more with a suspected or confirmed infection need aggressive treatment including.
- Investigations:
  - Complete blood count: There may be raised or low total leukocyte count
  - Lactate: Serum lactate levels especially lactate clearance has been found to have prognostic value in patients with septic shock[1]
  - Coagulation studies: Septic shock may be associated with coagulopathy.

- C-reactive protein: High value indicates inflammation. High CRP is commonly associated with sepsis.
- Procalcitonin: Elevated procalcitonin levels have been associated with sepsis and may help differentiate sepsis from causes of the systemic inflammatory response syndrome.[47]
- Workup to find source of infection if sepsis is suspected like blood cultures, urine culture, sputum culture and imaging like CXR, CT chest to exclude pneumonia or other intra-thoracic pathology, USG, CT scan of abdomen to locate any intra-abdominal source, etc.

Treatment of Septic Shock

- Resuscitate the patient, using supportive measures like oxygen to correct hypoxia, fluid and vasopressors for hypotension and hypoperfusion.
- Start appropriate empirical antibiotic therapy according to possible source of infection as soon as possible along with source control measures like incision drainage for abscess.
- Maintain adequate mean arterial pressure to improve tissue hypoperfusion and prevent progress to multiple organ dysfunction syndrome (MODS). Fluid administration should be continued as long as hemodynamic improvement continues.[48] Hemodynamic improvement is defined as increased organ perfusion, decreasing serum lactate and metabolic acidosis, and improved end-organ function. A sustained rise of more than 5 mm Hg in cardiac filling pressure after a fluid volume is infused indicates adequate filling and increased susceptibility to volume overload with further fluid administration. Administer vasopressors for hypotension that does not respond to initial fluid resuscitation to maintain a mean arterial pressure (MAP) of 65 mm Hg or higher. The recommended first-line agent for septic shock is norepinephrine. Vasopressin and adrenaline are included among the second-line agents. Corticosteroids (hydrocortisone) should be considered only for patients with vasopressor-dependent septic shock.

REFERENCES

1. Richards JB, Wilcox SR. Diagnosis and management of shock in the emergency department. Emerg Med Pract. 2014 Mar;16(3):1–22; quiz 22-3. PMID: 24883457.
2. Graham CA, Parke TR. Critical care in the emergency department: shock and circulatory support. Emerg Med J. 2005 Jan;22(1):17–21. doi: 10.1136/emj.2003.012450. PMID: 15611535; PMCID: PMC1726515.
3. Doerschug KC, Schmidt GA. Shock: Diagnosis and Management. In: Oropello JM, Pastores SM, Kvetan V. eds. Critical Care. McGraw Hill.
4. O'Brien C, Beaubien-Souligny W, Amsallem M, Denault A, Haddad F. Cardiogenic shock: reflections at the crossroad between perfusion, tissue hypoxia, and mitochondrial function. Canadian Journal of Cardiology. 2020 Feb 1; 36 (2): 184–96.
5. Bereda, Gudisa. (2021). Shock: Pathophysiology, Stage, Classification, and Treatment. Pathology and Laboratory Medicine. 5. 50–55. 10.11648/j.plm.20210502.16.
6. Boyan CP. Hypovolemic shock. Anesth Analg. 1967;46(6):746–750.
7. Schumer W. Hypovolemic shock. JAMA. 1979;241(6):615–616.
8. Shoemaker WC. Cardiorespiratory patterns in complicated and uncomplicated septic shock: physiologic alterations and their therapeutic implications. Ann Surg. 1971;174(1):119–125.
9. Romero-Bermejo FJ, Ruiz-Bailen M, Gil-Cebrian J, et al. Sepsis-induced cardiomyopathy. Curr Cardiol Rev. 2011;7(3):163–183.
10. Hackel DB, Ratliff NB, Mikat E. The heart in shock. Circ Res. 1974;35(6):805–811.
11. Rutherford RB, Hurt HH Jr, Brickman RD, et al. The patho-physiology of progressive, tension pneumothorax. J Trauma. 1968;8(2):212–227.

12. el Etr AA, Salem MR. Circulatory embarrassment in patients with large diaphragmatic hernias. Anesthesiology. 1968;29(1):164–165.
13. Podbregar M, Krivec B, Voga G. Impact of morphologic characteristics of central pulmonary thromboemboli in massive pulmonary embolism. Chest. 2002;122(3):973–979.
14. Doerschug KC, Schmidt GA. Shock: Diagnosis an Management. In: Oropello JM, Pastores SM, Kvetan V. eds. Critical Care. McGraw Hill.
15. Bonanno FG. Clinical pathology of the shock syndromes. J Emerg Trauma Shock. 2011 Apr;4(2):233–43.
16. Resuscitation Council (UK). Resuscitation guidelines: the ABCDE approach. 2021 [internet publication].
17. Rise IR, Kirkeby OJ. Effect of cerebral ischaemia on the cerebrovascular and cardiovascular response to haemorrhage. Acta Neurochir (Wien). 1998;140 (7):699–705.
18. Ibanez B, James S, Agewall S, et al. 2017 ESC Guidelines for the management of acute myocardial infarction in patients presenting with ST-segment elevation: The Task Force for the management of acute myocardial infarction in patients presenting with ST-segment elevation of the European Society of Cardiology (ESC). Eur Heart J. 2018 Jan 7;39 (2):119–77.
19. Chioncel O, Parissis J, Mebazaa A, et al. Epidemiology, pathophysiology and contemporary management of cardiogenic shock: a position statement from the Heart Failure Association of the European Society of Cardiology. Eur J Heart Fail. 2020 Aug;22(8):1315–41.
20. National Institute for Health and Care Excellence. Acute heart failure: diagnosis and management. Nov 2021.
21. [Guideline] O'Gara PT, Kushner FG, Ascheim DD, et al, for the American College of Cardiology Foundation/American Heart Association Task Force on Practice Guidelines. 2013 ACCF/AHA guideline for the management of ST-elevation myocardial infarction: a report of the American College of Cardiology Foundation/American Heart Association Task Force on Practice Guidelines. Circulation. 2013 Jan 29. 127 (4):e362–425.
22. Evans L, Rhodes A, Alhazzani W, et al. Surviving sepsis campaign: international guidelines for management of sepsis and septic shock 2021. Intensive Care Med. 2021 Nov;47(11):1181–247.
23. McDonagh TA, Metra M, Adamo M, et al. 2021 ESC guidelines for the diagnosis and treatment of acute and chronic heart failure. Eur Heart J. 2021 Sep 21;42(36):3599–726.
24. Wong SC, Sanborn T, Sleeper LA, Webb JG, Pilchik R, Hart D, Mejnartowicz S, Antonelli TA, Lange R, French JK, Bergman G, LeJemtel T, Hochman JS. Angiographic.
25. Holger Thiele, E. Magnus Ohman, Steffen Desch, Ingo Eitel, Suzanne de Waha, Management of cardiogenic shock, European Heart Journal, Volume 36, Issue 20, 21 May 2015, Pages 1223–1230.
26. National Institute for Health and Care Excellence. Acute heart failure: diagnosis and management. Nov 2021 [internet publication].
27. de Asua I, Rosenberg A. On the right side of the heart: medical and mechanical support of the failing right ventricle. J Intensive Care Soc. 2017; 18:113–120.
28. Cecconi M, De Backer D, Antonelli M, et al. Consensus on circulatory shock and hemodynamic monitoring: task force of the European Society of Intensive Care Medicine. Intensive Care Med. 2014 Dec;40(12):1795–815.
29. Baliga RR. Management of cardiogenic shock: AHA scientific statement. October 6, 2017.
30. Ouweneel DM, Henriques JPS. Percutaneous cardiac support devices for cardiogenic shock: current indications and recommendations. Heart. 2012; 98:1246–1254.
31. Abrams D, Combes A, Brodie D. Extracorporeal Membrane Oxygenation in Cardiopulmonary Disease in Adults. J Am Coll Cardiol 2014;63:2769–78.
32. Le Gall A, Follin A, Cholley B, et al. Veno-arterial-ECMO in the intensive care unit: From technical aspects to clinical practice. Anaesth Crit Care Pain Med 2018;37:259–68.
33. Garatti A, Russo C, Lanfranconi M, Colombo T, Bruschi G, Trunfio S, et al. Mechanical circulatory support for cardiogenic shock complicating acute myocardial infarction: an experimental and clinical review. ASAIO J. 2007 May-Jun. 53(3):278–87.
34. Cheng JM, den Uil CA, Hoeks SE, van der Ent M, Jewbali LS, van Domburg RT, et al. Percutaneous left ventricular assist devices vs. intra-aortic balloon pump counterpulsation for treatment of cardiogenic shock: a meta-analysis of controlled trials. Eur Heart J. 2009 Sep. 30(17):2102–8.

35. Windecker S. Percutaneous left ventricular assist devices for treatment of patients with cardiogenic shock. Curr Opin Crit Care. 2007 Oct. 13(5):521–7.
36. Hunt BJ, Allard S, Keeling D, et al. A practical guideline for the haematological management of major haemorrhage. Br J Haematol. 2015 Jul 6;170(6):788–803.
37. Lee JW. Fluid and electrolyte disturbances in critically ill patients. Electrolyte Blood Press. 2010 Dec;8(2):72–81.
38. MacLeod JB, Lynn M, McKenney MG, et al. Early coagulopathy predicts mortality in trauma. J Trauma. 2003 Jul;55(1):39–44.
39. Marik PE, Monnet X, Teboul JL. Hemodynamic parameters to guide fluid therapy. Ann Intensive Care. 2011;1(1):1.
40. Marik PE, Cavallazzi R. Does the central venous pressure predict fluid responsiveness? An updated metaanalysis and a plea for some common sense. Crit Care Med. 2013;41(7):1774–1781.
41. Miller A, Mandeville J. Predicting and measuring fluid responsiveness with echocardiography. Echo Res Pract. 2016 Jun;3(2):G1–12.
42. Kasotakis G, Sideris A, Yang Y, et al. Aggressive early crystalloid resuscitation adversely affects outcomes in adult blunt trauma patients: an analysis of the Glue Grant database. J Trauma Acute Care Surg. 2013;74(5):1215–1221.
43. Neal MD, Hoffman MK, Cuschieri J, et al. Crystalloid to packed red blood cell transfusion ratio in the massively transfused patient: when a little goes a long way. J Trauma Acute Care Surg. 2012;72(4):892–898.
44. Ley EJ, Clond MA, Srour MK, et al. Emergency department crystalloid resuscitation of 1.5 L or more is associated with increased mortality in elderly and nonelderly trauma patients. J Trauma. 2011;70(2):398–40.
45. Radwan ZA, Bai Y, Matijevic N, del Junco DJ, McCarthy JJ, Wade CE, Holcomb JB, Cotton BA. An emergency department thawed plasma protocol for severely injured patients. JAMA Surg. 2013 Feb;148(2):170-5. doi: 10.1001/jamasurgery.2013.414. PMID: 23426594; PMCID: PMC3800103.
46. Jennings LK, Watson S. Massive Transfusion. [Updated 2022 Aug 29]. In: StatPearls [Internet]. Treasure Island (FL): StatPearls Publishing; 2022 Jan.
47. Chalupa P, Beran O, Herwald H, et al. Evaluation of potential biomarkers for the discrimination of bacterial and viral infections. Infection. 2011 Oct;39(5):411–7.
48. Asfar P, Meziani F, Hamel JF, et al. High versus low blood-pressure target in patients with septic shock. N Engl J Med. 2014 Apr 24. 370(17):1583–93.

CHAPTER

7

Subarachnoid Hemorrhage
(Sudden Bleeding into the Subarachnoid Space)

Jorge Hidalgo, Barnabe Carrillo, Ahsina Jahan Lopa, Allyson Hidalgo

ABSTRACT

The presence of blood into the subarachnoid space, know as subarachnoid hemorrhage (SAH), is related to many etiologies. However, the most common cause is related with brain trauma involving all groups of age. We will review the primary causes of SAH as a result of the release of blood into the subarachnoid space most commonly due to a rupture of an aneurysm rupture. The secondary causes are most related to the leakage of blood products from intracerebral hemorrhage either directly into the subarachnoid space or via the ventricular system.

▪ **Keywords:** *Bleeding, subarachnoid space, malformation, headache.*

A 20-year-old male patient, rushed to emergency room, complaining of a sudden headache rated 10/10 and he described as one of the worst pains he ever had in life along with a brief loss of consciousness.

PMH: KNDA, Get severe COVID-19 in May, 2020, he was admitted in hospital for 4 weeks. Fully vaccinated for COVID-19.

Smokes and drinks alcohol occasionally.

His blood pressure was 190/98 mmHg, HR: 82, RR: 12. No fever SpO_2 at RA: 98%. Neurologic examination is unremarkable. We start him on IV fluids, pain control and BP control and soon he was more stable, we send him to have a brain CAT scan done without contrast and the radiologist described: Diffuse subarachnoid hemorrhage, mild brain swelling.

What are the next steps in the management of this patient?

What are the primary causes? Signs and symptoms?

What are common imaging findings?

Objectives of treatment? Rebleeding? Vasospasm?

What are some common subarachnoid haemorrhage etiologies?

The most common area of spontaneous SAH occurs in the circle of Willis, most commonly at the bifurcation of the middle cerebral artery. As a result of the rupture of a berry aneurysm or arteriovenous malformation, the risk increased by a history of high blood pressure. The most frequent location of a berry aneurysm is the anterior communicating artery, then the posterior communicating artery, followed by the middle cerebral artery. Trauma is the most common cause of SAH.[1]

▪ **Key point:** *Trauma is the most common cause of SAH.*

Primary Causes

1. Aneurysm
2. Arteriovenous malformation (AVM).

Less Common Causes are

1. Infectious aneurysms
2. Primary metastatic or meningeal neoplasms
3. Dural AVMs
4. Cavernous or venous angiomas
5. Nonstructural abnormalities include bleeding diathesis, iatrogenic coagulopathies, and systemic infections.[1,2]

Risk Factors

A few risk factors for SAH has been proposed:

1. Genetic predisposition
2. When two first-degree relatives have known aneurysm, it would appear reasonable to screen other close relatives.
3. Long-term exposure to smoking
4. Short-term exposure to alcohol
5. Vasoactive drugs like cocaine.[1,2]

Signs and Symptoms

Identifying patients at risk is critical in reducing morbidity and mortality. An average of 50% of the patients with a diagnosis of SAH die within 48 hours, irrespective of the therapy.

The most common description is to have an unusual headache, sudden headache (the worst headache in the patient's life), thunderclap headache. One important thing to mention is that the headache in SAH is not always noted as sudden, either because the patient does not perceive it that way or because the physician does not get the information. And a very intense headache, with photosensitivity; unconsciousness, even in a significant group of patients, does not awaken; neck pain, nuchal rigidity, photophobia, nausea, and vomiting.

- **Key point:** *The most common description is an unusual headache "the worst headache in the patient's life"*

The patients can also experience a sentinel headache, which can occur days or weeks before the rupture of the aneurysm. It could be the presentation of minor bleeding, a warning leak, or changes within the wall of the aneurysm.[3]

At the physical exam, we can encounter a patient with meningismus, the elevation of the blood pressure, preretinal hemorrhages (Terson syndrome), and signs of a poor prognosis. And the neurological findings are not specific, and it depends on the location of the bleeding, if hydrocephalus is present or not, increase in intracranial pressure, ischemic events, areas of infarction, or hematomas.

Involvement of pupil changes like third nerve palsy is frequently associated with SAH. It is often related to an expanding but not yet ruptured posterior communicating artery or superior cerebellar artery aneurysm close to where the third nerve exits the brainstem. If we have this finding, we need to proceed with the workup for an aneurysm.

- **Key point:** *One predictor of poor outcome is the presence of seizure in the initial 24 hours.*

Three common errors that can delay the diagnosis of SAH:

1. Proper interpretation of the medical history and clinical presentation.
2. Proper interpretation of the brain CAT scan, including the limitation in the diagnosis of SAH.
3. The decision to perform a lumbar puncture and finding the correct interpretation.

The presence of a murmur on cardiac examination is characteristic of mitral valve prolapse, which is commonly seen in Marfan's syndrome. The presence of berry aneurysm has been associated with Marfan's syndrome, Ehrlers-Danlos syndrome, adult polycystic kidney disease, and coarctation of the aorta.

Imaging Approach

One of the first steps is to obtain a non-contrast brain CAT scan (Figs 7.1 to 7.3).

Angiography over the year has been the GOLD standard test for diagnosing SAH. However, another imaging option has been gaining a place as an option, like a contrasted-enhanced brain CAT scan is an option. And also, we have brain Angio-MRI (Figs 7.4 to 7.8).

What are the typical findings of a cerebrospinal fluid analysis?

If the early brain CAT scan is negative for blood, then a lumbar puncture is mandatory if there is strong suspicious of SAH.

The cerebrospinal fluid in the SAH is usually bloody with a xanthochromia (hemoglobin degradation products) or yellow supernatant, a reflection of bilirubin release from the breakdown of hemoglobin—elevating opening pressure.[5]

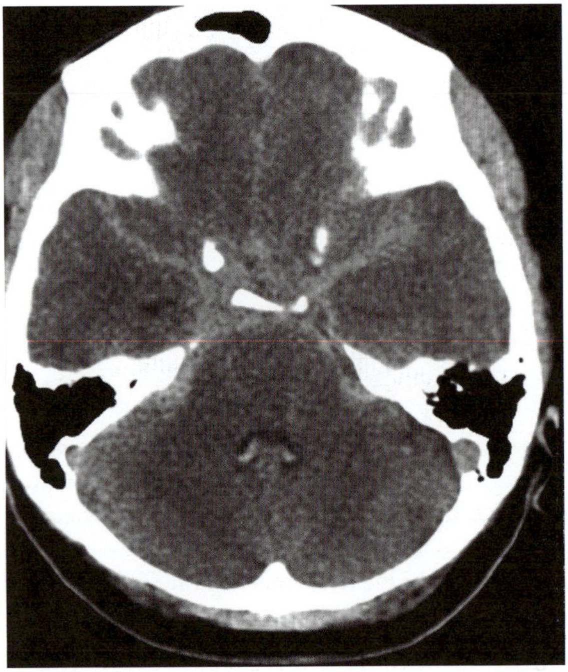

Fig. 7.1: Non-enhanced CT shows the presence of subarachnoid hemorrhage in the basal cisterns. Imaging is courtesy of: Far Eastern Memorial Hospital, New Taipei, Taiwan. Dr Yen-Jun Lai. Neuroradiologist. Dr Barnabe Carrillo, Interventional Neuroradiology Fellow.

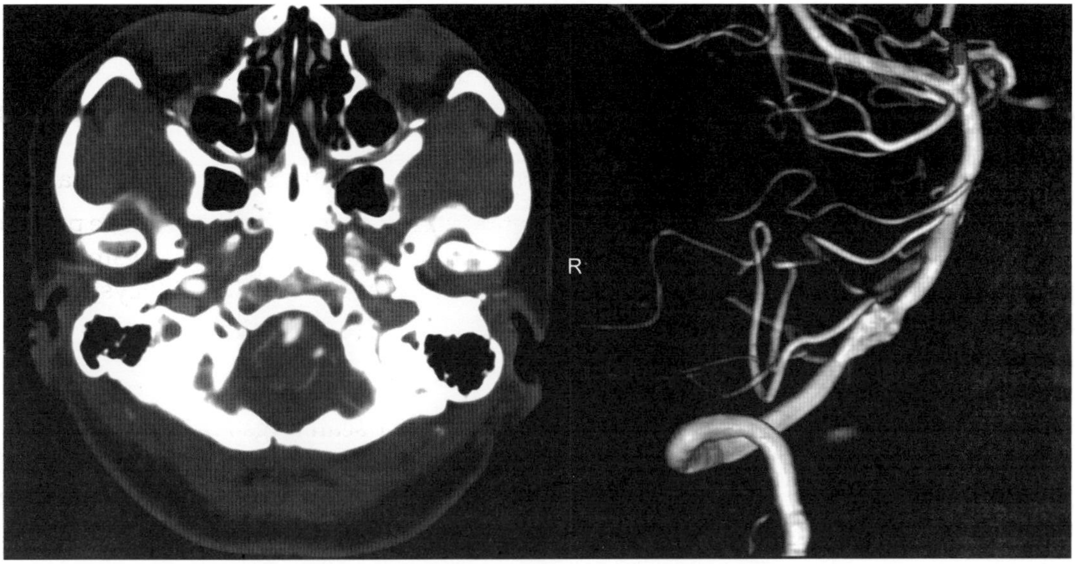

Fig. 7.2: CT angiography shows the source of the SAH to be a right vertebral artery (V4 segment) ruptured dissecting aneurysm confirmed on 3D angiography and treated successfully by neurointervention. Imaging is courtesy of: Far Eastern Memorial Hospital, New Taipei, Taiwan. Dr Yen-Jun Lai. Neuroradiologist. Dr Barnabe Carrillo, Interventional Neuroradiology Fellow.

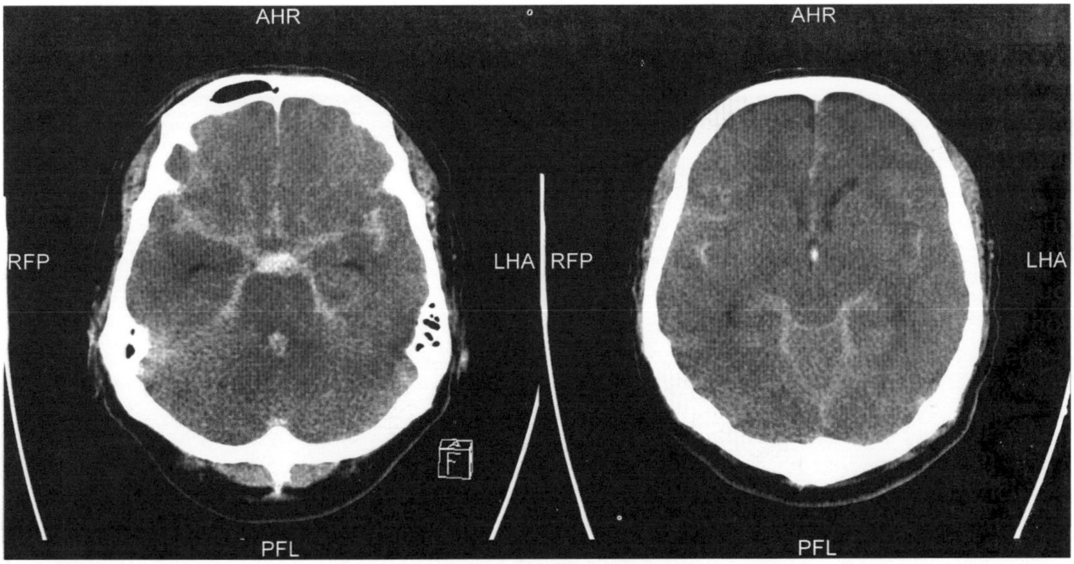

Fig. 7.3: Non-enhanced CT shows diffuse SAH in the basal cisterns, bilateral cerebral and cerebellar convexities and intraventricular (fourth ventricle) hemorrhage due to a fusiform aneurysm of the left Vertebral artery (V4 segment). Imaging is courtesy of: Far Eastern Memorial Hospital, New Taipei, Taiwan. Dr Yen-Jun Lai. Neuroradiologist. Dr Barnabe Carrillo, Interventional Neuroradiology Fellow.

Most common complication of SAH are rebleeding, hydrocephalus, cerebral edema, vasospasm and delayed cerebral ischemia and seizures. Metabolic complication, like electrolyte disturbances mainly hyponatremia and neuroendocrine dysfunction.[5]

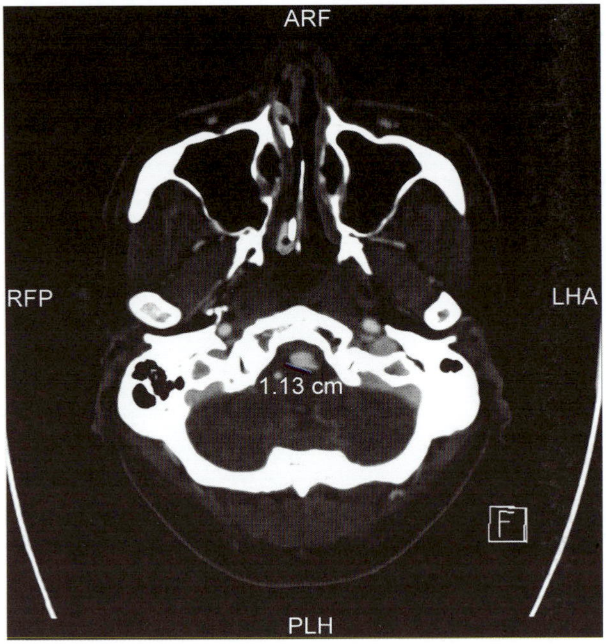

Fig. 7.4: CT angiography shows a fusiform aneurysm of the left V4 segment of the vertebral artery. Imaging is courtesy of: Far Eastern Memorial Hospital, New Taipei, Taiwan. Dr Yen-Jun Lai. Neuroradiologist. Dr Barnabe Carrillo, Interventional Neuroradiology Fellow.

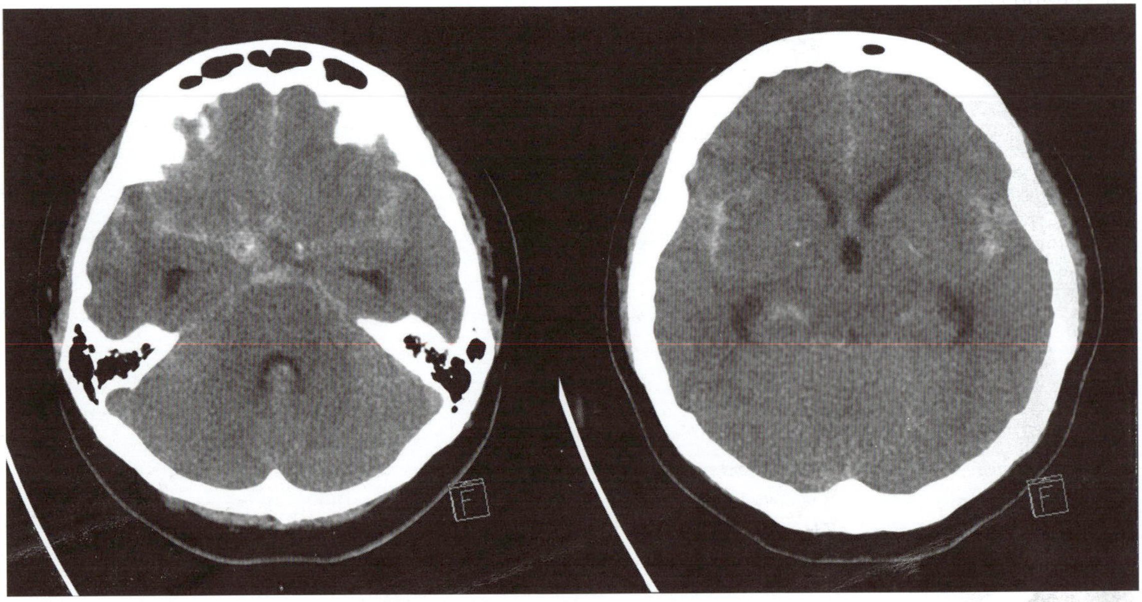

Fig. 7.5: Non-enhanced CT shows diffuse subarachnoid hemorrhage in the basal cisterns, bilateral sylvian fissures and cerebral sulci, due to suspected internal carotid artery aneurysm. Note dilatation of the temporal horns of the lateral ventricles and third ventricle. Imaging is courtesy of: Far Eastern Memorial Hospital, New Taipei, Taiwan. Dr Yen-Jun Lai. Neuroradiologist. Dr Barnabe Carrillo, Interventional Neuroradiology Fellow.

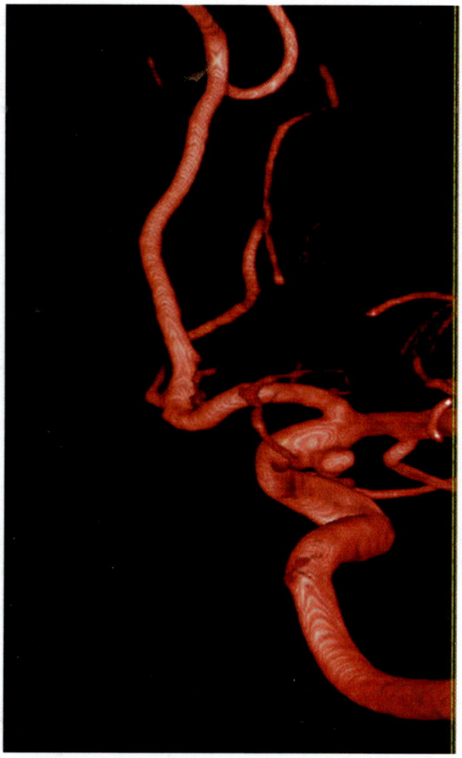

Fig. 7.6: 3D rotational angiography shows the presence of a 3 mm anterior choroidal artery aneurysm in the right internal carotid artery. Imaging is courtesy of: Far Eastern Memorial Hospital, New Taipei, Taiwan. Dr Yen-Jun Lai. Neuroradiologist. Dr Barnabe Carrillo, Interventional Neuroradiology Fellow.

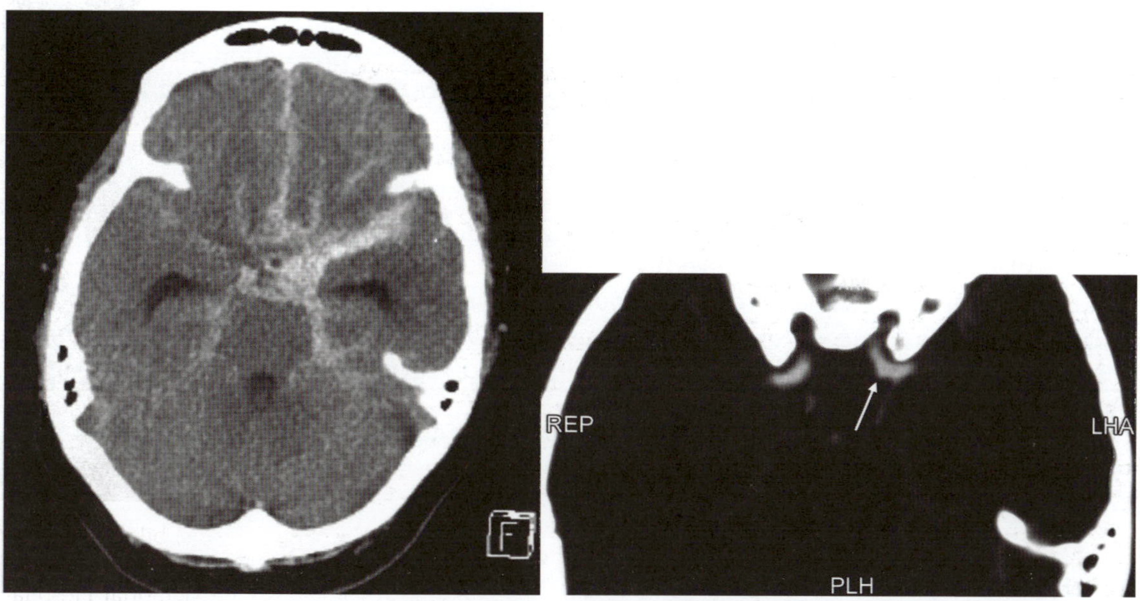

Fig. 7.7: Non-enhanced CT shows subarachnoid hemorrhage with bleeding concentrated mostly in the left basal cisterns and left sylvian fissure. This was due to a blister aneurysm seen on the CT angiography Image.

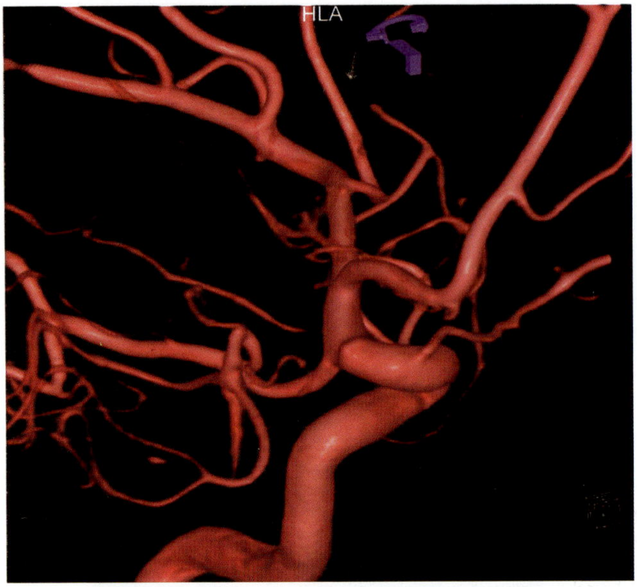

Fig. 7.8: Rotational 3D angiography confirms diagnosis of a blister aneurysm in the dorsomedial aspect of the left supraclinoid internal carotid artery. Patient was treated successfully with a flow diverter. Imaging is courtesy of: Far Eastern Memorial Hospital, New Taipei, Taiwan. Dr Yen-Jun Lai. Neuroradiologist. Dr Barnabe Carrillo, Interventional Neuroradiology Fellow.

Treatment

The first step is the stabilization of the patient, addressing any life-threatening conditions, especially in those patients in coma. Ensuring and secure airway, normalizing the cardiovascular function, and control the seizures.[7]

The most important point is to identify and to eliminate the causative lesion and preventing rebleeding. The second point is to treat hydrocephalous and a critical part is to preventing and treating the vasospasm. And another critical component is the prevention or identification of hydrocephalus. Hence is crucial, a proper managed of the Spinal Cerebral Fluid (SCF) volume and any obstruction of the CSF dynamics.[6,7]

Admission or transfer the patient to a more resource facility.

Blood pressure control.

Discontinuation or reversal of all anticoagulants, until the aneurysm is treated either by surgery or minimally invasive procedure.

Antifibrinolytic agents should not be routinely used in SAH.

DVT prophylaxis needs to start with mechanic devices like, intermittent pneumatic compression devices and chemoprophylaxis can be added in any modality once the aneurysm has been treated properly.

Proper management of the IV fluids (euvolemia maintenance)

Proper monitorization with any available modality:

- Transcranial Doppler.
- Brain and vascular imaging
- Continuous electroencephalography
- Regular neuro-evaluation and monitoring studies
- Intracranial pressure monitoring.[7]

Vasospasm: As soon as the patient is stable within the 48 hours periods of the diagnosis of SAH, we need to start with Nimodipine, a calcium channel blocker, the recommended dosage is 60 mg every four hours, either orally or by nasogastric tube and we need to continue for 21 days. The exact mechanism of benefit of Nimodipine in SAH is unknown.[1,7]

Final Points

- Subarachnoid haemorrhage (SAH) is a neurologic emergency.
- A sudden severe headache is one of the most common clinical presentations.
- Patient with SAH should be evaluating immediately and coordinate admission to ICU.
- Patient with SAH can experiences several complications among others: Hydrocephalus, rebleeding, seizures, electrolytes disorders mainly sodium disorders.
- As soon as possible we need to implement vasospasm strategies prophylaxis.

REFERENCES

1. Edlow JA, Caplan LR. Avoiding pitfalls in the diagnosis of subarachnoid hemorrhage. N Engl J Med 2000; 342:29.
2. Perry JJ, Stiell IG, Sivilotti ML, et al. High risk clinical characteristic for subarachnoid haemorrhage in patients with acute headache: Prospective cohort study. BMJ 2010; 342:c540.
3. Polmear A. Sentinel headaches in aneurysmal subarachnoid haemorrhage: what is the true incidence? A systematic review. Cephalagia 2003; 23:935.
4. Michael T Lawton, Vates. Subarachnoid Hemorrhage. N Engl J Med 2017; 377:257–266.
5. Saeedi, Morteza, et al. "Determining the Value of Cerebrospinal Fluid Lactate Dehydrogenase Level in Differentiating Subarachnoid Hemorrhage From Traumatic Lumbar Puncture." Archives of Pathology & Laboratory Medicine, vol. 142, no. 5, College of American Pathologists, May 2018, p. 634.
6. Van Gijn J, Kerr RS, Rinkel GJ. Subarachnoid haemorrhage. Lancet 2007; 369:306.
7. Robert J Singer, Christopher S Ogilvy, Guy Rordorf. Aneurysm Subarachnoid Hemorrhage: Treatment and prognosis. UpToDate. December 06, 2022.

CHAPTER

8

ARDS

Javier Perez-Fernandez, Paola Perez

A 46-year-old man was evaluated at the emergency department with increased shortness of breath, cough, and low-grade temperature for two days. He was seen by his primary physician the day before and was prescribed symptomatic-relief treatment for his cold-related symptoms. Because of worsening progression, he presented to our hospital. Upon evaluation he was noted pale, with increased respiratory muscle retraction and with an oxygen saturation of 82%. His chest radiograph is shown in Fig. 8.1. He was immediately given oxygen via nasal cannula at 5 L/min and broad-spectrum antibiotics, macrolide and a penicillin/beta-lactamase inhibitor agent, were rapidly started. Within the following hours the clinical deterioration was notorious and soon the patient had to be placed in high-flow nasal cannula at 100% while maintaining only marginal oxygen saturations (88–91%). Admitted to the intensive care unit, he failed an attempt of non-invasive ventilation and was intubated shortly thereafter. A CT scan of the chest was performed (Fig. 8.2). The clinical diagnosis was ARDS secondary to pneumonia. Initial ventilator settings were chosen according to ARDS-net recommendations, with a tidal volume calculated at 5 mL/kg/PBW. His plateau pressures were 28 cm H_2O while he required 10 cm H_2O of PEEP to maintain adequate oxygenation. The

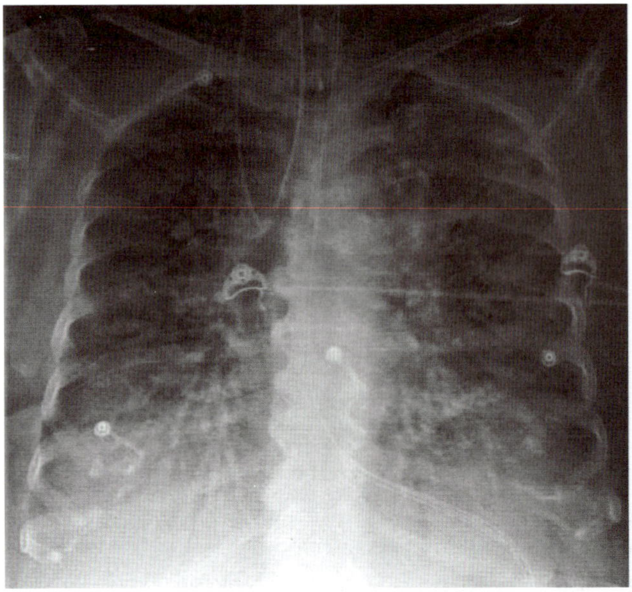

Fig. 8.1: Chest radiograph

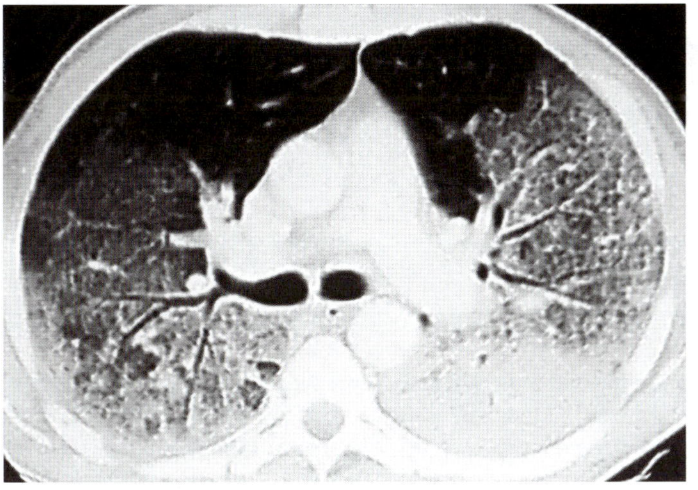

Fig. 8.2: Chest CT scan

patient was ventilated while maintaining lung protective strategies for the following days. BAL samples were negative for bacteria, but serology was indicative of acute mycoplasma infection. The patient continued with progressive improvement and was extubated 74 hours after the intubation being finally discharged from the hospital 5 days later.

ARDS DEFINITIONS

Acute (or adult) respiratory distress syndrome (ARDS) is characterized by the inflammatory response of the lungs to a direct or indirect insult. Pneumonia, trauma, aspiration, sepsis, or pancreatitis are some of the conditions associated to the development of ARDS.[1] Although no definitive pathophysiologic mechanism has been stablished, there is direct injury to the alveolar cells, surfactant alteration, immune system activation and dysregulation of the blood clotting system.[2,3,4]

Formally described in 1967, affects over three million people worldwide annually.[5] In the nineteen seventies and eighties, multiple studies showed varied outcomes, high mortality and perhaps related to the lack of uniformity in the criteria, a disparity in management recommendations. In 1994 the first American-European Consensus Conference was held in Berlin, and it was the origin of the first definitions.[6] Since then, a more standardized process and guidance for studies and management exist.

Pathophysiology

Multiple risk factors have been identified in the etiology of ARDS.[2,3,4] It is unknown why some patients with those conditions progress to the development of ARDS versus others do not. The lung injury prediction score (LIPS) aims to incorporate known risk factors to predict the likelihood to develop ARDS.[7]

Although all these were an attempt to grade and classify ARDS, they lack insight into the pathophysiology of the development of ARDS. The mechanisms of ARDS are complex and involves the dysregulation of multiple interacting pathways of injury, inflammation, and coagulation, not only at the lung level but also systemically.

The classic pathological feature is diffuse alveolar damage. The presence of hyaline membranes, alveolar hemorrhagic features and fibrin deposits accompanied with endothelial injury are characteristic although not universally present.[4,8] Injury to the lung's epithelial and endothelial barriers is responsible for the increased capillary leak and for the abnormalities in gas exchange.[9] Alveolar flooding is responsible for gas exchanges abnormalities while disrupting the surfactant lining and inducing alveolar collapse. This forces the affected individual to exercise higher inspiratory pressures and increased work of breathing. Microvascular thromboses and damage to vascular bed may be contributing factors for vascular changes (pulmonary hypertension and ventricular dysfunction) and dead space ventilation.[10,11]

Systemic Inflammation

In the early phases of ARDS, there is migration of neutrophils to the alveolar spaces inducing a release of pro-inflammatory substances (prostaglandins and leukotrienes) and mediators such as interleukins.[12,13] There is increasing evidence that lymphocytes and dendritic cells are also involved in the inflammatory response.[14] The presence of systemic injury in patients with ARDS can be attributed in part to the release of all these inflammatory elements.

An additional factor came to play in the last two decades: The recognition of mechanical ventilation as an independent contributor of lung injury. Volutrauma (or Volume Induced Lung Injury: VILI) and barotrauma are the resultant of the application of positive pressure (and volumes) to the heterogeneous lung areas of the affected lung. The concept of 'baby lung' has come to explain this phenomenon.[15] In addition, those areas are confronted to repeated shear forces in the opening and closing faces, the fact that is enhanced by the disruption and ineffectiveness in the surfactant, a concept defined as atelectrauma.[16]

Classification and Phenotyping

Classically, ARDS has been divided into mild, moderate, and severe according to the oxygen level of the patients or the PaO_2/FiO_2 ratio. (200 to 300 mmHg, 100 to 200 mmHg and <100 mm Hg). More recently, phenotyping ARDS has called the attention of the academic and clinical community. Phenotyping could improve our understanding of ARDS pathophysiology and help us to modify outcomes.[17] Predictive enrichment might potentially impact risk reduction in some populations in clinical trials, thus improving our clinical application in some others.

COVID-19 enhanced the topic of phenotyping even more, as we realized that some patients presented varied radiologic features that reflected into different clinical presentations and outcomes.[18] Physiological variants with differential responses to lung recruitment maneuvers may also be an important factor in ARDS. Some patients might be presenting increased dead space ventilation, whereas some other might demonstrate more recruitable areas of alveoli.[19]

There are also differences in pulmonary and extrapulmonary ARDS, being the latest more prone to express more endothelial and a more diffuse pattern of injury.[20] Cause-specific ARDS has also been part of research. Transfusion-related ARDS and trauma among others have not only been studied in their relation to the development of ARDS but also on regards to interventions aimed to decrease their incidence.[21,22]

Different inflammatory phenotypes have also been described. Some studies have associated the presence of hyperinflammation with extrapulmonary sepsis and a worse prognostic indicator, although the former has not been fully demonstrated.[23,24]

MANAGEMENT

Lung Protective Strategies

The most important advance in the management of ARDS patients was the adoption of limited-low-volume ventilation following the findings of the ARMA trial.[25] Avoiding over distension of the lung during mechanical ventilation of ARDS patients is called lung protective ventilation (LPV). LPV, with volumes below 6 mL/kg of predicted body weight, while maintaining a plateau pressure (Pp) less than 30 cm of H_2O has become the standard treatment to provide mechanical ventilation to patients with ARDS. The calculation of predicted body weight is based on height, according to the formulas:

$$\text{Male IBW(kg)} = 50 + 0.91\ (\text{cm height} - 152.4)$$
$$\text{Female IBW (kg)} = 45.5 + 0.91\ (\text{cm height} - 152.4)$$

Recently attention has been directed to driving pressure as an independent variable for prognosis in patients with ARDS. Driving pressure, calculated as the difference between Pp and PEEP has correlated well, as a sole factor, with increased mortality.[26,27] Mechanical power, which is the energy per unit time released to the respiratory system, a factor calculated based on delivered tidal volume, PEEP, respiratory rate, and flow, is associated with lung injury and is recently being subject of increasing research.[28] It is remarkable to mention that there is lack of large prospective trials analyzing results of reduction of driving pressures or mechanical power, thus although the growing evidence suggest the need for controlling both during ventilation in patients with ARDS, no standard recommendations can be made.

Pressure-limited ventilation has been widely used to ventilate patients and has the intrinsic benefit to limit the plateau pressure to a desired value. However, its impact on mortality or other aspects of ventilated patients with ARDS has not been demonstrated.[29,30]

Non-standard ventilatory methods can provide benefit when applied to individual patients under singular circumstances. The use of APRV or bilevel ventilation allows spontaneous breathing and has been postulated that could prevent respiratory muscle weakness.[31]

Non-ventilatory Interventions

Proning

The PROSEVA trial demonstrated that proning patients18 hours per day resulted in mortality benefit.[32] The COVID 19 pandemic has impulse the use of proning, both in ventilated and non-ventilated patients presenting with COVID-related ARDS (C-ARDS), an entity that was soon to be differentiated from non-COVID ARDS.[33,34] The benefit of proning for C-ARDS seem not to be directly related to improvements in lung compliance, raising the possibility of differentiated phenotypes in patients with C-ARDS and the need for alternate treatments according to such phenotypes.[35]

A separate mention deserves the use of proning in awake, non-intubated, patients, a practice that became extensively popular during the pandemic. Small observational studies and a randomized trial demonstrated 28-day mortality improvement in patients with C-ARDS.[36]

ECMO

In a recent trial in the UK, ECMO was associated to mortality benefit in ARDS.[37] However, mortality benefit was also observed by the clustering of patients into an ECMO referral center, whether ECMO was or not applied. Multiple small series and case reports were published during the pandemic. The current evidence suggests that ECMO can improve oxygenation in refractory ARDS, but its outcomes might be dependent on its application in experienced in its use.

Neuromuscular Blockade

Current sedation practices are ultimately guided by the Society of Critical Care Medicine's PADIS guidelines.[38] Neuromuscular blockade and its mortality benefit continues to be a topic of study. ACURASYS trial showed 90-day mortality benefit with early (within 48 hours) neuromuscular blockade.[39] However, the more recent ROSE trial, showed no mortality benefit between light sedation with neuromuscular blockade and early deep sedation, although noted that deep sedatives caused some more ventilator asynchrony.[40]

Corticosteroids

The use of corticosteroids in the treatment of patients with ARDS has been a long-standing controversy. The ARDS Network performed the largest trial to date examining whether corticosteroids benefit ARDS patients.[41] Although no mortality benefit was ultimately achieved, there was a trend in favorable outcomes, included ventilator-free days and patient-days alive in early start of steroids as opposed to a contrary effect in those who were started after day 14 of the diagnosis. Although the recommendations continue being diverse, if the decision is to use corticosteroids, it is recommended to do it within the first two weeks. In addition, clinicians should exercise special attention to glucose control and caution with steroid-enhanced muscle weakness. The effect of the steroids in prolonging viral replication in viral-related ARDS has not been demonstrated and the benefit of this therapy was well-established in C-ARDS.[42]

CONCLUSIONS

Our case was illustrative of community acquired pneumonia that progressed rapidly to ARDS. The mechanisms to differentiate why some patients progress rapidly to ARDS, whereas others do not are to be cleared. Phenotyping might be the answer and as our knowledge becomes deeper in this element, we might be able to target characteristics of those patients. Much we learnt in the management of ARDS patients within the last two decades. The single most important factor to decrease mortality is the use of protective lung ventilation. More than twenty years after adopting these measures, and with strong evidence support, there is a concerning lack of adherence to this practice worldwide.[43] Other treatment strategies are being considered, but any impact derived from those, is only seen when added to the protective strategies.

REFERENCES

1. Marino, Paul (2006). The ICU Book. Baltimore: Williams & Wilkins. ISBN 978-0781748025.
2. Bellani G, Laffey JG, Pham T et al. Epidemiology, patterns of care, and mortality for patients with acute respiratory distress syndrome in intensive care units in 50 countries. JAMA. 2016; 315: 788–800Vvv
3. Matthay MA, Zemans RL, Zimmerman GA, et al. Acute respiratory distress syndrome. Nat Rev Dis Primers. 2019; 5:18.
4. Thille AW, Peñuelas O, Lorente JA, et al. Predictors of diffuse alveolar damage in patients with acute respiratory distress syndrome: a retrospective analysis of clinical autopsies. Crit Care. 2017; 21: 254.
5. Ashbaugh DG, Bigelow DB, Petty TL, Levine BE. Acute respiratory distress in adults. Lancet. 1967; 2: 319–323.
6. Ranieri VM, Rubenfeld GD, Thompson BT, et al; ARDS Definition Task Force. Acute respiratory distress syndrome: the Berlin Definition. JAMA. 2012;307(23):2526–2533.
7. Gajic O, Dabbagh O, Park PK, Adesanya A, Chang SY, Hou P, Anderson H 3rd, Hoth JJ, Mikkelsen ME, Gentile NT, Gong MN, Talmor D, Bajwa E, Watkins TR, Festic E, Yilmaz M, Iscimen R, Kaufman DA, Esper AM, Sadikot R, Douglas I, Sevransky J, Malinchoc M, U.S. Critical Illness and Injury Trials Group: Lung Injury Prevention Study Investigators (USCIITG-LIPS): Early identification of patients at risk of acute lung injury: Evaluation of lung injury prediction score in a multicenter cohort study. Am J Respir Crit Care Med 2011; 183:462–70.

8. Thille AW, Esteban A, Fernández-Segoviano P, et al. Comparison of the Berlin definition for acute respiratory distress syndrome with autopsy. Am J Respir Crit Care Med. 2013; 187: 761–767.
9. Nuckton TJ, Alonso JA, Kallet RH, et al. Pulmonary dead-space fraction as a risk factor for death in the acute respiratory distress syndrome. N Engl J Med. 2002; 346: 1281–1286.
10. Petit M, Jullien E, Vieillard-Baron A. Right ventricular function in acute respiratory distress syndrome: impact on outcome, respiratory strategy and use of veno-venous extracorporeal membrane oxygenation. Front Physiol. 2022; 12797252.
11. Nuckton TJ, Alonso JA, Kallet RH, et al. Pulmonary dead-space fraction as a risk factor for death in the acute respiratory distress syndrome. N Engl J Med. 2002; 346: 1281–1286.
12. Lin WC, Fessler MB. Regulatory mechanisms of neutrophil migration from the circulation to the airspace. Cell Mol Life Sci. 2021; 78: 4095–4124.
13. Lefrançais E, Mallavia B, Zhuo H et al. Maladaptive role of neutrophil extracellular traps in pathogen-induced lung injury. JCI Insight. 2018; 398178.
14. Perl M, Lomas-Neira J, Venet F, et al. Pathogenesis of indirect (secondary) acute lung injury. Expert Rev Respir Med. 2011; 5: 115–126.
15. Gattinoni L, Presenti A. The concept of "baby lung". Intensive Care Med. 2005; 31: 776–784.
16. Muscedere JG, Mullen JBM, Gan K, et al. Tidal ventilation at low airway pressures can augment lung injury. Am J Respir Crit Care Med. 1994; 149: 1327–1334.
17. Ware LB, Matthay MA, Mebazaa A. Designing an ARDS trial for 2020 and beyond: focus on enrichment strategies. Intensive Care Med. 2020; 46: 2153–2156.
18. Boss LDJ, Sjouding M, Sinha P et al. Longitudinal respiratory subphenotypes in patients with COVID-19-related acute respiratory distress syndrome: results from three observational cohorts. Lancet Respir Med. 2021; 9: 1377–1386.
19. Wendel Garcia PD, Cacciopola A, Copola S, et al. Latent class analysis to predict intensive care outcomes in acute respiratory distress syndrome: a proposal of two pulmonary phenotypes. Crit Care. 2021; 25: 154.
20. Pelosi, P, D'Onofrio D, Chiumello D, et al. Pulmonary and extrapulmonary acute respiratory distress syndrome are different. Eur Respir J Suppl. 2003; 42: 48s–56s.
21. Eder AF, Herron Jr RM, Strupp A, et al. Effective reduction of transfusion-related acute lung injury risk with male-predominant plasma strategy in the American Red Cross (2006–2008). Transfusion. 2010; 50: 1732–1742.
22. Li G, Malinchoc M, Cartin-Ceba R, et al. Eight-year trend of acute respiratory distress syndrome: a population-based study in Olmsted County, Minnesota. Am J Respir Crit Care Med. 2011; 183: 59–66.
23. Calfee CS, Delucchi K, Parsons PE, et al. Subphenotypes in acute respiratory distress syndrome: latent class analysis of data from two randomised controlled trials. Lancet Respir Med. 2014; 2: 611–620.
24. Sinha P, Delucchi KL, Thompson BT, et al. Latent class analysis of ARDS subphenotypes: a secondary analysis of the statins for acutely injured lungs from sepsis (SAILS) study. Intensive Care Med. 2018; 44: 1859–1869.
25. The Acute Respiratory Distress Syndrome Network. Ventilation with lower tidal volumes as compared with traditional tidal volumes for acute lung injury and the acute respiratory distress syndrome. N Engl J Med. 2000;342(18):1301–1308.
26. Amato MBP, Meade MO, Slutsky AS, Brochard L, Costa ELV, Schoenfeld DA, et al. Driving pressure and survival in the acute respiratory distress syndrome. N Engl J Med. 2015;372(8):747–55.
27. Baedorf Kassis E, Loring SH, Talmor D. Mortality and pulmonary mechanics in relation to respiratory system and transpulmonary driving pressures in ARDS. Intensive Care Med. 2016;42(8):1206–13.
28. Coppola S, Caccioppola A, Froio S, Formenti P, De Giorgis V, Galanti V, Consonni D, Chiumello D. Effect of mechanical power on intensive care mortality in ARDS patients. Crit Care. 2020 May 24;24(1):246.
29. Marini JJ. Point: Is pressure assist-control preferred over volume assist-control mode for lung protective ventilation in patients with ARDS? Yes. Chest 2011;140:286.
30. Chacko B, Peter JV, Tharyan P, John G, Jeyaseelan L. Pressure-controlled versus volume-controlled ventilation for acute respiratory failure due to acute lung injury (ALI) or acute respiratory distress syndrome (ARDS). Cochrane Database Syst Rev. 2015 Jan 14;1(1):CD008807. doi: 10.1002/14651858.CD008807.pub2. PMID: 25586462; PMCID: PMC6457606.

31. Tobin MJ, Franco Laghi F, Jubran A. Narrative Review: Ventilator-Induced Respiratory Muscle Weakness. Ann Int Med 2010;153:240–245.
32. Guérin C, Reignier J, Richard JC, Beuret P, Gacouin A, Boulain T, Mercier E, Badet M, Mercat A, Baudin O, Clavel M, Chatellier D, Jaber S, Rosselli S, Mancebo J, Sirodot M, Hilbert G, Bengler C, Richecoeur J, Gainnier M, Bayle F, Bourdin G, Leray V, Girard R, Baboi L, Ayzac L, PROSEVA Study Group. Prone positioning in severe acute respiratory distress syndrome.N Engl J Med 2013;368:2159.
33. Panwar, R., Madotto, F., Laffey, J., & van Haren, F. (2020). Compliance Phenotypes in Early Acute Respiratory Distress Syndrome before the COVID-19 Pandemic. American Journal Of Respiratory And Critical Care Medicine, 202(9), 1244-1252. doi: 10.1164/rccm.202005-2046oc
34. Gattinoni, L., & Marini, J. (2021). Isn't it time to abandon ARDS? The COVID-19 lesson. Critical Care, 25(1). doi: 10.1186/s13054-021-03748–6.
35. Gattinoni, L., Chiumello, D., Caironi, P., Busana, M., Romitti, F., Brazzi, L., & Camporota, L. (2020). COVID-19 pneumonia: different respiratory treatments for different phenotypes?. Intensive Care Medicine, 46(6), 1099-1102. doi: 10.1007/s00134-020-06033–2.
36. Kaur, R., Vines, D., Mirza, S., Elshafei, A., Jackson, J., & Harnois, L. et al. (2021). Early versus late awake prone positioning in non-intubated patients with COVID-19. Critical Care, 25(1). doi: 10.1186/s13054-021-03761–9.
37. Peek GJ, Mugford M, Tiruvoipati R, Wilson A, Allen E, Thalanany MM, Hibbert CL, Truesdale A, Clemens F, Cooper N, Firmin RK, Elbourne D, CESAR trial collaboration. Lancet Efficacy and economic assessment of conventional ventilatory support versus extracorporeal membrane oxygenation for severe adult respiratory failure (CESAR): a multicentre randomised controlled trial. Lancet 2009;374(9698):1351.
38. Devlin, J., Skrobik, Y., Gélinas, C., Needham, D., Slooter, A., & Pandharipande, P. et al. (2018). Clinical Practice Guidelines for the Prevention and Management of Pain, Agitation/Sedation, Delirium, Immobility, and Sleep Disruption in Adult Patients in the ICU. Critical Care Medicine, 46(9), e825–e873.
39. Papazian L, Forel JM, Gacouin A, Penot-Ragon C, Perrin G, Loundou A, Jaber S, Arnal JM, Perez D, Seghboyan JM, Constantin JM, Courant P, Lefrant JY, Guérin C, Prat G, Morange S, Roch A Neuromuscular blockers in early acute respiratory distress syndrome. ACURASYS Study Investigators. N Engl J Med 2010;363:1107.
40. The National Heart, Lung and Blood Institute PETAL Clinical Trial Network. Early Neuromuscular Blockade in the Acute Respiratory Distress Syndrome. (2019). New England Journal Of Medicine, 380(21), 1997–2008. doi: 10.1056/nejmoa1901686.
41. Steinberg KP, Hudson LD, Goodman RB, Hough CL, Lanken PN, Hyzy R, Thompson BT, Ancukiewicz M, National Heart, Lung, and Blood Institute Acute Respiratory Distress Syndrome (ARDS) Clinical Trials Network Efficacy and safety of corticosteroids for persistent acute respiratory distress syndrome. N Engl J Med 2006;354:1671.
42. RECOVERY Collaborative Group, Horby P, Lim WS, et al. Dexamethasone in hospitalized patients with COVID-19. N Engl J Med. 2021;384(8):693–704.
43. Weiss CH, Baker DW, Weiner S, et al. Low tidal volume ventilation use in acute respiratory distress syndrome. Crit Care Med. 2016; 44:1515–1522.

CHAPTER

9

Management of Sepsis

Carlos Sanchez

CASE PRESENTATION

A 48-year-old male, with no history of illness, not taking any medication, apparently healthy, who lives in the countryside and works as a farmer, came to the emergency department because 3 days ago while working he injured the skin around his navel with a plant that it had thorns but he extracted the thorn with his fingers, that same night he started with erythema in said area, the skin was also hot and general malaise, during those three days the skin became hard, with a red-brown color, headache, thirst, weakness, his wife decides to medicate him with a topical antibiotic and ibuprofen but the next day he was taken to the hospital because the lesions worsened, at the time of admission the patient was sleepy, he reported feeling bad, he had not urinated since the day before, HR 119, RR 28, SpO_2 95% room air, temp 38.6°C, BP 86/52 mmHg. On physical examination, the mucous membranes are dry, capillary refill time 5 sec, and the following skin lesions are found:

What Approach should Guide this Septic Patient?

Since sepsis and septic shock are emergencies, the mortality rates of these patients can reach as high as 60% even with current recommended treatments. That is why these patients should be adequately cared for immediately in the place where they are diagnosed and, as soon as possible, be transferred to a health center where there are personnel trained in the management of this type of patient and, if possible, have an intensive care unit.

Although there are some guidelines worldwide on how these patients should be managed, there is no consensus on all aspects of therapy. What is certain is that these patients progress to multiple organ failure, the longer it takes to restore hemodynamic stability and the longer the microorganisms remain in the host body, which is why the main pillars in the management of patients with sepsis and septic shock are mainly based on the use of fluids, vasopressors and antibiotics.

This patient was received in the emergency department, an intravenous bolus of fluids 500 ml balanced solution was administered over 15 min, immediately he was admitted to the ICU where norepinephrine was started until reaching a MAP of 65–70 mmHg, after that 500 ml more of fluid IV were administered, cultures of the skin lesion and blood cultures were taken, treatment was started with vancomycin 1 gm IV q 12 h + clindamycin 600 mg IV q 8h thinking of cellulitis complicated with fasciitis caused by *Staphylococcus aureus*. The patient evolves favorably during the first 24 hours and is taken to the operating room by general surgery to perform surgical cleaning of the lesions, but after that there is a greater need for norepinephrine, reaching a dose of 0.42 µg/kg/min. He started with hydrocortisone

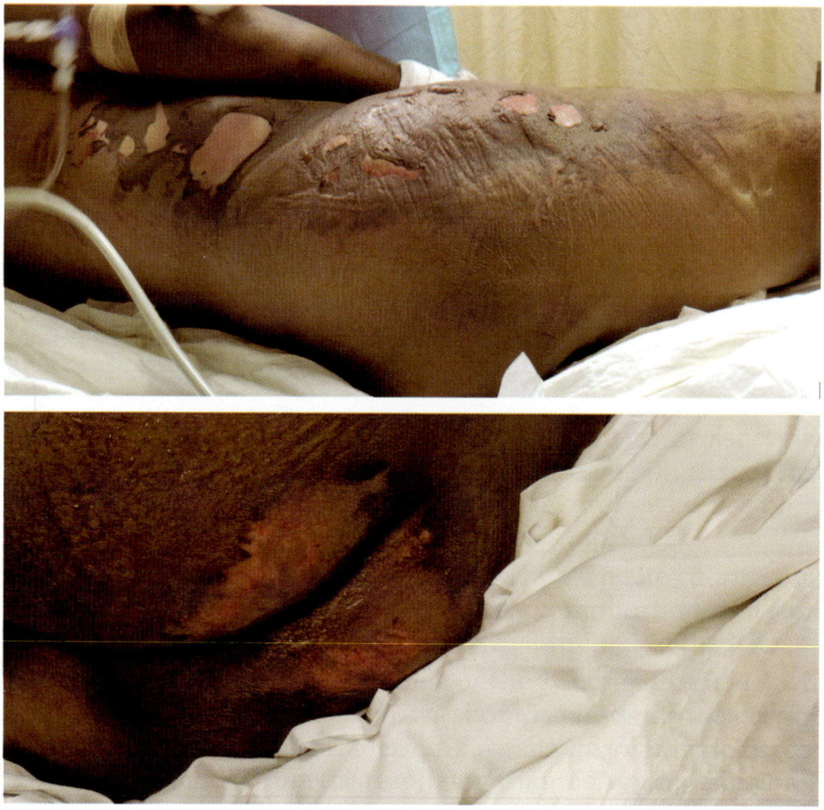

Fig. 9.1: Bacterial infection of the skin growth of *E. coli*

100 mg IV stat and then 50 mg q 6 h, in addition to starting IV vasopressin at 0.02 IU/h, diuresis improved 3 h later. After 24 hours, growth of *E. coli* was reported in the culture of the skin secretion and meropenem 1 g IV q 8 h was added, 36 h after starting this medication, hemodynamics began to improve, it was possible to discontinue vasopressin and decrease the dose of norepinephrine, until 5 days later discontinuation was achieved, the patient received control of source management of the lesion every 48 h and 11 days later he was discharged alive from the ICU to the general surgery hospital ward.

PRINCIPLES OF MANAGEMENT

Diagnosis: There is not any score or laboratory test accepted worldwide to diagnose sepsis, so suspicion will be the first approach to diagnosis. Although the most accurate diagnosis of sepsis is based on clinical symptoms, biomarkers and microbiology, there are some internationally proposed scales for initial suspicion and possibility of complications, including the qSOFA and SOFA score.[1]

1. **qSOFA:** The patient with documented or highly suspected infection must meet at least 2 of the following 3 variables: Glasgow Coma Scale <13, Systolic Blood Pressure <100 mmHg and Respiratory Rate > 22 (Table 9.1).[1] This score is usually applied as the first guiding assessment in the first contact with the patient, but it should not be used as the only tool to diagnose sepsis.[2]
2. **SOFA:** Patient with documented or highly suspected infection and the presence of at least 2 new points on the SOFA scale (Table 9.2) with respect to the baseline level.[1]

Table 9.1: qSOFA Score/Criteria

qSOFA (quick SOFA) criteria	*Points*
Respiratory rate ≥22/min	1
Change in mental status	1
Systolic blood pressure ≤100 mmHg	1

Table 9.2: Sequential organ failure assessment score

Organ system	*Score*				
	0	*1*	*2*	*3*	*4*
Respiratory PaO_2/FiO_2	≥400 mmHg (53.3 kPa)	<400 mmHg (53.3 kPa)	<300 mmHg (40 kPa)	<200 mmHg (26.7 kPa) with respiratory support	<100 mmHg (13.3 kPa) with respiratory support
Coagulation platelets	≥150 × 10^3/µL	<150	<100	<50	<20
Hepatic bilirubin	<1.2 mg//dL (20 µmol/L)	1.2–1.9 mg/dL (20–32 µmol/L)	2.0–5.9 mg/dL (33–101 µmol/L)	6.0–11.9 mg/dL (102–204 µmol/L)	>12 mg/dL (204 µmol/L)
Cardiovascular MAP	≥70 mmHg	<70	Dopamine <5 µg/kg per minute or any dose of dobutamine	Dopamine 5.1–15 µg/ kg per minute or epineprine ≤0.1 µg/kg per minute or norepinephrine ≤0.1 µg/kg per minute	Dopamine >15 or epinephrine >0.1 or norepineprine >0.1
Central nervous system: Glasgow Coma Scale score	15	13–14	10–12	6–9	<6
Renal	Serum creatinine <12 mg/dL (110 µmol/L)	Serum creatinine 1.2–1.9 mg/dL (110–170 µmol/L)	Serum creatinine 2.0–3.4 mg/dL (171–299 µmol/L)	Serum creatinine 3.5–4.9 mg/dL (300–440 µmol/L) or urine output <500 mL/d	Serum creatinine >5.0 mg/dL (440 µmol/L) or urine output <200 mL/d

FiO_2 fraction of inspired oxygen; MAP, mean arterial pressure; PaO_2, partial pressure of oxygen.

In order to diagnose the state of septic shock, in addition to these sepsis criteria, the patient must have arterial hypotension that does not improve with fluids alone and therefore requires vasopressors, as well as microcirculation alteration, which can be followed by elevation of serum lactate or by refill capillary time >3 sec.[3] In both criteria, the need for vasopressors and impaired tissue perfusion must be present to make the diagnosis.[1]

Hemodynamic stabilization: This point includes two aspects: Macro and microhemodynamics, firstly the efforts are aimed at stabilizing macrohemodynamics, mainly blood pressure, MAP, heart rate and secondly microhemodynamics, capillary refill time, mottling score, SvO_2, delta CO_2, thermal gradient among others.[4]

To achieve this hemodynamic stability, we have two main strategies: Fluids and vasopressors.

Fluids: There are currently two main strategies for fluid management, liberal[2,5] and restrictive.[6,7] Based on the current evidence, it has been possible to demonstrate how harmful the administration of large amounts of fluids is, the repercussion on the different organs and systems and, of course, the negative impact that this causes on the mortality of patients.[8–12] On the other hand, fluid restriction seems to be a strategy that is not inferior to standard management and that leads to a reduction in the number of organic failures as well as an improvement in the existing ones.[7] Understanding that patients with septic shock do not have real hypovolemia but vasodilation, the administration of fluids must be very well justified, and it should only be administered if this leads to intravascular volume stress, for which the accepted strategy is after giving an initial bolus of crystalloids and seeing if there is hemodynamic improvement, this maneuver does not require further monitoring as long as there is no great risk of heart failure or fluid overload.[13] After the initial bolus, maneuvers such as passive lifting of the legs to assess whether it is responsive to fluid administration.[14]

The response to fluids is a reflex that wears out over time, therefore it is important to determine the time that the patient has been in septic shock, since at the moment the state of shock is established, only approximately 70% of patients they respond to the administration of fluids and after 2 hours only approximately 25% will respond, reaching less than 10% after 4 hours.[15]

Another important aspect about the administration of fluids is the infusion time, this should be infused in a time of 10–30 min, shorter times could lead to heart failure or pulmonary edema and longer times could increase the compliance of the blood vessels,[16] allow leakage into the interstitial tissue and thus not achieving the expected volume stress.[12]

Vasopressors: In septic shock, what occurs mainly at the hemodynamic level is sustained vasodilatation, which leads to the subtype of vasoplegic shock.[17] Restoring vascular tone is the main priority in septic shock patients, this is achieved by using vasopressors as soon as possible, this can be before, during and in some cases after fluid administration.[2] It has been shown that mortality increases directly the longer the administration of vasopressors is delayed,[18] since arterial hypotension is a determinant of mortality, not only the degree of arterial hypotension but also the time of hypotension.[17]

The vasopressor of choice is norepinephrine. If the expected response is not achieved, another preferably non-catecholamine vasopressor such as vasopressin, angiotensin II, among others, can be associated.[2]

If it is decided to administer a vasopressor, its administration should not be delayed, and it is recommended to start via the peripheral route if the patient does not have a central venous catheter.[2]

Antibiotics: Not all cases of septic shock are caused by bacteria, so not all patients need antibiotics. In some cases, infections are caused by fungi and antifungals should be given,[2] in other cases by viruses or parasites and here the therapeutic options are scarcer.

Empirical antibiotic therapy should be directed at the possible causative agent according to the patient's symptoms or according to the sensitivity shown in the antibiogram if there is one.[2] For patients in septic shock, it seems more reasonable to use two antibiotics and for septic patients without shock, a single antibiotic could be sufficient for most cases, with some exceptions when multi-resistant germs are involved.[2,19]

For patients with septic shock, the administration of antimicrobials should not necessarily be the priority, since in them hemodynamic stabilization is the priority. There are studies that have found that there is no difference in terms of mortality with respect to the time of administration of antimicrobials in patients with septic shock, first 3 hours or after that period.[20,21]

Control of the infectious focus: Although this has been known since ancient medical practices, it has not been until recent years that special importance has been given to the control/removal of the focus, finding in recent studies that this practice is carried out by experienced hands and in the right moment leads to a significant increase in the chances of survival, mainly in patients with intra-abdominal and soft tissue infections.[22] It is important to stabilize the patient before submitting him to any type of surgical intervention, times less than 2 hours to perform the removal appear to be associated with increased mortality.[23] However, whenever possible, surgical removal of the infectious focus should be scheduled.

Supportive care: No less important is keeping the patient adequately nourished, guaranteeing their active and passive mobilization, as far as possible allowing family visits while maintaining isolation measures according to the germ, using strategies aimed at reducing delirium.

Advanced life support: If the patient presents with organ failure that requires advanced support such as renal replacement therapy, ECMO, mechanical ventilation (with a protective ventilation strategy, if necessary) should be provided without any contraindication.

EVIDENCE CONTOUR

There are still many debatable aspects in the management of septic patients, ranging from the measurement of serum lactate to the use of interleukin removal as part of the advanced management of sepsis. Below we will try to mention the most debated strategies in a timely manner.

Measurement of serum lactate: Serum lactate rises under stress conditions without this signifying tissue hypoxia.[24] The beta-adrenergic stimulation of patients in great stress or in those who use catecholamines, mainly adrenaline, may present high levels of lactate, beyond this, elevated serum lactate only predicts the higher mortality, which lowers the probability of survival.[25]

Taking blood cultures: Approximately 80–90% of patients who come to the hospital with sepsis have negative blood cultures,[26] regardless of whether or not they have been receiving antibiotics.[27] Most international management guidelines suggest that blood cultures be taken before starting antimicrobials,[2] if changes are made to them, or if the patient worsens, but there is no evidence to support improved survival by taking blood cultures, it is best to take cultures of possibly infected fluids or tissues whenever possible without delaying administration of antimicrobials.

Steroids: Treatment with physiological doses of hydrocortisone for 5 to 7 days increases survival and resolution of shock in patients with vasopressor-dependent septic shock. Currently there are some schemes regarding its use without demonstrating that one is superior to the others, the two most recommended are hydrocortisone at a dose of 50 mg IV q 6 h or 200 mg in continuous infusion for 24 h. However, treatment with high doses of glucocorticoids for a short course decreases the survival of patients with sepsis.[2,28]

Vitamin C and thiamine: This therapy was proposed by Dr Marik as part of a cocktail in which vitamin C 1.5 gm IV q6 h was associated for 4 days or until discharge from the ICU, thiamine 100 mg IV q 12 h, and hydrocortisone.[29,30] Although it is true that there are some small studies that report improvement in patients, so far there is no conclusive evidence that the use of this therapy can help improve patients in septic shock.[31]

Methylene blue: It represents a non-adrenergic vasopressor with limited effectiveness in patients with refractory distributive shock. The development of profound tissue hypoxia and a high degree of anaerobic metabolism was associated with the loss of hemodynamic responsiveness to its administration. In patients with refractory shock receiving methylene blue, there is a non-statistically significant trend towards improved outcomes in responders based on a MAP increase >10%. Patients supported with CRRT who were identified as responders had decreased ICU mortality compared to non-responders.[32]

The optimal dose is unknown, but the most commonly used dose is 1–2 mg/kg in a bolus or infusion over 1 hour.

Hemoperfusion: Although it is not a new therapy, it has only been during the COVID-19 pandemic that it has taken off worldwide. Sepsis is a syndrome in which the main problem is immunological dysregulation,[1] therefore, it is totally reasonable to think that removing these immunological substances from the blood (interleukins, NTF, etc.), patients should improve. However, it must maintain a balance of pro-inflammatory and anti-inflammatory substances,[33] but this type of therapy is not selective and removes both types. The SSC 2021 guidelines consider that there is currently insufficient evidence to make a pronouncement regarding hemoperfusion techniques in sepsis.[2] The little evidence is very heterogeneous with studies that report that mortality worsens, others that it is not affected, and others that say that it improves.[34] Perhaps it is still necessary to better identify the patient who could benefit from said therapy, when, how long and perhaps the type of device to be used.[35]

REFERENCES

1. Singer M, Deutschman CS, Seymour CW, et al. The Third International Consensus Definitions for Sepsis and Septic Shock (Sepsis-3). *JAMA*. 2016;315(8):801–810. doi:10.1001/jama.2016.0287
2. Evans L, Rhodes A, Alhazzani W, Antonelli M, Coopersmith CM, French C, Machado FR, Mcintyre L, Ostermann M, Prescott HC, Schorr C, Simpson S, Wiersinga WJ, Alshamsi F, Angus DC, Arabi Y, Azevedo L, Beale R, Beilman G, Belley-Cote E, Burry L, Cecconi M, Centofanti J, Coz Yataco A, De Waele J, Dellinger RP, Doi K, Du B, Estenssoro E, Ferrer R, Gomersall C, Hodgson C, Møller MH, Iwashyna T, Jacob S, Kleinpell R, Klompas M, Koh Y, Kumar A, Kwizera A, Lobo S, Masur H, McGloughlin S, Mehta S, Mehta Y, Mer M, Nunnally M, Oczkowski S, Osborn T, Papathanassoglou E, Perner A, Puskarich M, Roberts J, Schweickert W, Seckel M, Sevransky J, Sprung CL, Welte T, Zimmerman J, Levy M. Surviving sepsis campaign: international guidelines for management of sepsis and septic shock 2021. Intensive Care Med. 2021 Nov;47(11):1181–1247. doi: 10.1007/s00134-021-06506-y. Epub 2021 Oct 2. PMID: 34599691; PMCID: PMC8486643.
3. Hernández G, Ospina-Tascón GA, Damiani LP, Estenssoro E, Dubin A, Hurtado J, Friedman G, Castro R, Alegría L, Teboul JL, Cecconi M, Ferri G, Jibaja M, Pairumani R, Fernández P, Barahona D, Granda-Luna V, Cavalcanti AB, Bakker J; The ANDROMEDA SHOCK Investigators and the Latin America Intensive Care Network (LIVEN), Hernández G, Ospina-Tascón G, Petri Damiani L, Estenssoro E, Dubin A, Hurtado J, Friedman G, Castro R, Alegría L, Teboul JL, Cecconi M, Cecconi M, Ferri G, Jibaja M, Pairumani R, Fernández P, Barahona D, Cavalcanti AB, Bakker J, Hernández G, Alegría L, Ferri G, Rodriguez N, Holger P, Soto N, Pozo M, Bakker J, Cook D, Vincent JL, Rhodes A, Kavanagh BP, Dellinger P, Rietdijk W, Carpio D, Pavéz N, Henriquez E, Bravo S, Valenzuela ED, Vera M, Dreyse J, Oviedo V, Cid MA, Larroulet M, Petruska E, Sarabia C, Gallardo D, Sanchez JE, González H, Arancibia JM, Muñoz A, Ramirez G, Aravena F, Aquevedo A, Zambrano F, Bozinovic M, Valle F, Ramirez M, Rossel V, Muñoz P, Ceballos C, Esveile

C, Carmona C, Candia E, Mendoza D, Sanchez A, Ponce D, Ponce D, Lastra J, Nahuelpán B, Fasce F, Luengo C, Medel N, Cortés C, Campassi L, Rubatto P, Horna N, Furche M, Pendino JC, Bettini L, Lovesio C, González MC, Rodruguez J, Canales H, Caminos F, Galletti C, Minoldo E, Aramburu MJ, Olmos D, Nin N, Tenzi J, Quiroga C, Lacuesta P, Gaudín A, Pais R, Silvestre A, Olivera G, Rieppi G, Berrutti D, Ochoa M, Cobos P, Vintimilla F, Ramirez V, Tobar M, García F, Picoita F, Remache N, Granda V, Paredes F, Barzallo E, Garcés P, Guerrero F, Salazar S, Torres G, Tana C, Calahorrano J, Solis F, Torres P, Herrera L, Ornes A, Peréz V, Delgado G, López A, Espinosa E, Moreira J, Salcedo B, Villacres I, Suing J, Lopez M, Gomez L, Toctaquiza G, Cadena Zapata M, Orazabal MA, Pardo Espejo R, Jimenez J, Calderón A, Paredes G, Barberán JL, Moya T, Atehortua H, Sabogal R, Ortiz G, Lara A, Sanchez F, Hernán Portilla A, Dávila H, Mora JA, Calderón LE, Alvarez I, Escobar E, Bejarano A, Bustamante LA, Aldana JL. Effect of a Resuscitation Strategy Targeting Peripheral Perfusion Status vs Serum Lactate Levels on 28-Day Mortality Among Patients With Septic Shock: The ANDROMEDA-SHOCK Randomized Clinical Trial. JAMA. 2019 Feb 19;321(7):654-664. doi: 10.1001/jama.2019.0071. PMID: 30772908; PMCID: PMC6439620.

4. Abele Donati, Roberta Domizi, Elisa Damiani, Erica Adrario, Paolo Pelaia, Can Ince. From Macrohemodynamic to the Microcirculatiom. Hindawi Publishing Corporation Critical Care Research and Practice Volume 2013, Article ID 892710, 8 pages http://dx.doi.org/10.1155/2013/892710
5. Emanuel Rivers, M.D., M.P.H., Bryant Nguyen, M.D., Suzanne Havstad, M.A., Julie Ressler, B.S., Alexandria Muzzin, B.S., Bernhard Knoblich, M.D., Edward Peterson, Ph.D., and Michael Tomlanovich, M.D. for the Early Goal-Directed Therapy Collaborative Group. Early Goal-Directed Therapy in the Treatment of Severe Sepsis and Septic Shock. November 8, 2001 N Engl J Med 2001; 345:1368-1377 DOI: 10.1056/NEJMoa010307
6. Hjortrup PB, Haase N, Bundgaard H, Thomsen SL, Winding R, Pettilä V, Aaen A, Lodahl D, Berthelsen RE, Christensen H, Madsen MB, Winkel P, Wetterslev J, Perner A; CLASSIC Trial Group; Scandinavian Critical Care Trials Group. Restricting volumes of resuscitation fluid in adults with septic shock after initial management: the CLASSIC randomised, parallel-group, multicentre feasibility trial. Intensive Care Med. 2016 Nov;42(11):1695-1705. doi: 10.1007/s00134-016-4500-7. Epub 2016 Sep 30. PMID: 27686349.
7. Hjortrup PB, Haase N, Wetterslev J, Lange T, Bundgaard H, Rasmussen BS, Dey N, Wilkman E, Christensen L, Lodahl D, Bestle M, Perner A. Effects of fluid restriction on measures of circulatory efficacy in adults with septic shock. Acta Anaesthesiol Scand. 2017 Apr;61(4):390–398. doi: 10.1111/aas.12862. Epub 2017 Feb 1. PMID: 28150304.
8. The ARISE Investigators and the ANZICS Clinical Trials Group. Goal-Directed Resuscitation for Patients with Early Septic Shock. N Engl J Med 2014; 371:1496–1506 DOI: 10.1056/NEJMoa1404380
9. Paul R. Mouncey, M.Sc., Tiffany M. Osborn, M.D., G. Sarah Power, M.Sc., David A. Harrison, Ph.D., M. Zia Sadique, Ph.D., Richard D. Grieve, Ph.D., Rahi Jahan, B.A., Sheila E. Harvey, Ph.D., Derek Bell, M.D., Julian F. Bion, M.D., Timothy J. Coats, M.D., Mervyn Singer, M.D., J. Duncan Young, D.M., and Kathryn M. Rowan, Ph.D. for the ProMISe Trial Investigators. Trial of Early, Goal-Directed Resuscitation for Septic Shock. N Engl J Med 2015; 372:1301–1311 DOI: 10.1056/NEJMoa1500896
10. ProCESS Investigators, Yealy DM, Kellum JA, Huang DT, Barnato AE, Weissfeld LA, Pike F, Terndrup T, Wang HE, Hou PC, LoVecchio F, Filbin MR, Shapiro NI, Angus DC. A randomized trial of protocol-based care for early septic shock. N Engl J Med. 2014 May 1;370(18):1683-93. doi: 10.1056/NEJMoa1401602. Epub 2014 Mar 18. PMID: 24635773; PMCID: PMC4101700.
11. The PRISM Investigators. Early, Goal-Directed Therapy for Septic Shock — A Patient-Level Meta-Analysis. N Engl J Med 2017; 376:2223-2234 DOI: 10.1056/NEJMoa1701380
12. Malbrain, M.L.N.G., Van Regenmortel, N., Saugel, B. et al. Principles of fluid management and stewardship in septic shock: it is time to consider the four D's and the four phases of fluid therapy. Ann. Intensive Care 8, 66 (2018). https://doi.org/10.1186/s13613-018-0402-x
13. Spiegel R. Stressed vs. unstressed volume and its relevance to critical care practitioners. Clin Exp Emerg Med. 2016 Mar 31;3(1):52-54. doi: 10.15441/ceem.16.128. PMID: 27752616; PMCID: PMC5051617.
14. Monnet, X., Teboul, JL. Passive leg raising: five rules, not a drop of fluid!. Crit Care 19, 18 (2015). https://doi.org/10.1186/s13054-014-0708-5
15. Silversides JA, Perner A, Malbrain MLNG. Liberal versus restrictive fluid therapy in critically ill patients. Intensive Care Med. 2019 Oct;45(10):1440-1442. doi: 10.1007/s00134-019-05713-y. Epub 2019 Aug 9. PMID: 31399779.

16. Toscani L, Aya HD, Antonakaki D, Bastoni D, Watson X, Arulkumaran N, Rhodes A, Cecconi M. What is the impact of the fluid challenge technique on diagnosis of fluid responsiveness? A systematic review and meta-analysis. Crit Care. 2017 Aug 4;21(1):207. doi: 10.1186/s13054-017-1796-9. PMID: 28774325; PMCID: PMC5543539.
17. Varpula M, Tallgren M, Saukkonen K, Voipio-Pulkki LM, Pettilä V. Hemodynamic variables related to outcome in septic shock. Intensive Care Med. 2005 Aug;31(8):1066–71. doi: 10.1007/s00134-005-2688-z. Epub 2005 Jun 23. PMID: 15973520.
18. Li Y, Li H, Zhang D. Timing of norepinephrine initiation in patients with septic shock: a systematic review and meta-analysis. Crit Care. 2020 Aug 6;24(1):488. doi: 10.1186/s13054-020-03204-x. PMID: 32762765; PMCID: PMC7409707.
19. Kumar A, Zarychanski R, Light B, Parrillo J, Maki D, Simon D, Laporta D, Lapinsky S, Ellis P, Mirzanejad Y, Martinka G, Keenan S, Wood G, Arabi Y, Feinstein D, Kumar A, Dodek P, Kravetsky L, Doucette S; Cooperative Antimicrobial Therapy of Septic Shock (CATSS) Database Research Group. Early combination antibiotic therapy yields improved survival compared with monotherapy in septic shock: a propensity-matched analysis. Crit Care Med. 2010 Sep;38(9):1773-85. doi: 10.1097/CCM.0b013e3181eb3ccd. PMID: 20639750.
20. Peltan ID, Brown SM, Bledsoe JR, Sorensen J, Samore MH, Allen TL, Hough CL. ED Door-to-Antibiotic Time and Long-term Mortality in Sepsis. Chest. 2019 May;155(5):938-946. doi: 10.1016/j.chest.2019.02.008. Epub 2019 Feb 16. PMID: 30779916; PMCID: PMC6533450.
21. Weinberger J, Rhee C, Klompas M. A Critical Analysis of the Literature on Time-to-Antibiotics in Suspected Sepsis. J Infect Dis. 2020 Jul 21;222(Suppl 2):S110-S118. doi: 10.1093/infdis/jiaa146. PMID: 32691835.
22. Reitz KM, Kennedy J, Li SR, Handzel R, Tonetti DA, Neal MD, Zuckerbraun BS, Hall DE, Sperry JL, Angus DC, Tzeng E, Seymour CW. Association Between Time to Source Control in Sepsis and 90-Day Mortality. JAMA Surg. 2022 Sep 1;157(9):817-826. doi: 10.1001/jamasurg.2022.2761. PMID: 35830181; PMCID: PMC9280613.
23. De Pascale G, Antonelli M, Deschepper M, Arvaniti K, Blot K, Brown BC, de Lange D, De Waele J, Dikmen Y, Dimopoulos G, Eckmann C, Francois G, Girardis M, Koulenti D, Labeau S, Lipman J, Lipovetsky F, Maseda E, Montravers P, Mikstacki A, Paiva JA, Pereyra C, Rello J, Timsit JF, Vogelaers D, Blot S; Abdominal Sepsis Study (AbSeS) group and the Trials Group of the European Society of Intensive Care Medicine. Poor timing and failure of source control are risk factors for mortality in critically ill patients with secondary peritonitis. Intensive Care Med. 2022 Nov;48(11):1593-1606. doi: 10.1007/s00134-022-06883-y. Epub 2022 Sep 23. PMID: 36151335.
24. Levy B, Desebbe O, Montemont C, Gibot S. Increased aerobic glycolysis through beta2 stimulation is a common mechanism involved in lactate formation during shock states. Shock. 2008 Oct;30(4):417-21. doi: 10.1097/SHK.0b013e318167378f. PMID: 18323749.
25. Casserly B, Phillips GS, Schorr C, Dellinger RP, Townsend SR, Osborn TM, Reinhart K, Selvakumar N, Levy MM. Lactate measurements in sepsis-induced tissue hypoperfusion: results from the Surviving Sepsis Campaign database. Crit Care Med. 2015 Mar;43(3):567-73. doi: 10.1097/CCM.0000000000000742. PMID: 25479113.
26. Sigakis MJG, Jewell E, Maile MD, Cinti SK, Bateman BT, Engoren M. Culture-Negative and Culture-Positive Sepsis: A Comparison of Characteristics and Outcomes. Anesth Analg. 2019 Nov;129(5):1300-1309. doi: 10.1213/ANE.0000000000004072. PMID: 30829670; PMCID: PMC7577261.
27. Previsdomini M, Gini M, Cerutti B, Dolina M, Perren A. Predictors of positive blood cultures in critically ill patients: a retrospective evaluation. Croat Med J. 2012 Feb 15;53(1):30-9. doi: 10.3325/cmj.2012.53.30. PMID: 22351576; PMCID: PMC3284177.
28. Keh D, Trips E, Marx G, Wirtz SP, Abduljawwad E, Bercker S et al. Effect of Hydrocortisone on Development of Shock Among Patients With Severe Sepsis: The HYPRESS Randomized Clinical Trial. JAMA 2016 Nov 1; 316(17):1775-1785.
29. Marik PE, Khangoora V, Rivera R, Hooper MH, Catravas J. Hydrocortisone, vitamin C and thiamine for the treatment of severe sepsis and septic shock: a retrospective before-after study. Chest 2017; 151(6):1229–1238.
30. Marik PE. Patterns of Death in Patients with Sepsis and the Use of Hydrocortisone, Ascorbic Acid, and Thiamine to Prevent These Deaths. Surg Infect (Larchmt) 2018; 19(8):812-820.

31. Fowler AA 3rd, Truwit JD, Hite RD, Morris PE, DeWilde C, Priday A, Fisher B, Thacker LR 2nd, Natarajan R, Brophy DF, Sculthorpe R, Nanchal R, Syed A, Sturgill J, Martin GS, Sevransky J, Kashiouris M, Hamman S, Egan KF, Hastings A, Spencer W, Tench S, Mehkri O, Bindas J, Duggal A, Graf J, Zellner S, Yanny L, McPolin C, Hollrith T, Kramer D, Ojielo C, Damm T, Cassity E, Wieliczko A, Halquist M. Effect of Vitamin C Infusion on Organ Failure and Biomarkers of Inflammation and Vascular Injury in Patients With Sepsis and Severe Acute Respiratory Failure: The CITRIS-ALI Randomized Clinical Trial. JAMA. 2019 Oct 1;322(13):1261-1270. doi: 10.1001/jama.2019.11825. Erratum in: JAMA. 2020 Jan 28;323(4):379. PMID: 31573637; PMCID: PMC6777268.
32. Porizka, Michal & Kopecky, Patrik & Dvorakova, Helena & Kunstyr, Jan & Lips, Michal & Michalek, Pavel & Balik, Martin. (2020). Methylene blue administration in patients with refractory distributive shock – a retrospective study. Scientific Reports. 10. 10.1038/s41598-020-58828-4.
33. Honore PM, Hoste E, Molnár Z, Jacobs R, Joannes-Boyau O, Malbrain MLNG, Forni LG. Cytokine removal in human septic shock: Where are we and where are we going? Ann Intensive Care. 2019 May 14;9(1):56. doi: 10.1186/s13613-019-0530-y. PMID: 31089920; PMCID: PMC6517449.
34. Wendel Garcia PD, Hilty MP, Held U, Kleinert EM, Maggiorini M. Cytokine adsorption in severe, refractory septic shock. Intensive Care Med. 2021 Nov;47(11):1334-1336. doi: 10.1007/s00134-021-06512-0. Epub 2021 Sep 1. PMID: 34471938; PMCID: PMC8409473.
35. Schultz P, Schwier E, Eickmeyer C, Henzler D, Köhler T. High-dose CytoSorb hemoadsorption is associated with improved survival in patients with septic shock: A retrospective cohort study. J Crit Care. 2021 Aug;64:184-192. doi: 10.1016/j.jcrc.2021.04.011. Epub 2021 Apr 20. PMID: 33962219.

CHAPTER 10

Shock and Hemodynamic Targets and Management

Tarun Kapoor, Lillie Pitts, Cassidy Vigil, Ashish K Khanna

CASE

A 65-year-old female with a medical history of poorly controlled diabetes (most recent hemoglobin A1C 9.5%), hypertension, heart failure with reduced ejection fraction (most recently 40–45%), and alcohol abuse was brought to the hospital when her husband found her minimally responsive in bed. According to her husband, she was complaining of nausea and a productive cough before he went to work and found her in bed on his return. He states that she has approximately 2–3 drinks a day with the most recent likely day before admission. Her most recent set of medications include metformin 1000 mg BID, empagliflozin 25 mg daily, losartan 50 mg daily, multiple ibuprofen a day, and lasix 40 mg every other day.

On arrival at the hospital, she is found to have a BP of 90/40, HR 110/min, RR 30/min, Temp of 39.5 Celsius, and GCS of 8 (2,2,4).

Initial Physical Exam

General: Lethargic, pale, ill-appearing woman

Head: Atraumatic, normocephalic

Neck: Supple, full ROM, no lymphadenopathy

Cardiovascular: Tachycardia, S1 S2 present, no murmurs, rubs, or gallops

Respiratory: Tachypneic, diffuse coarse breath sounds, decreased breath sounds over right lower lung fields increased work of breathing.

Abdomen: Soft, non-tender, non-distended

Extremities: Cool, palpable pulse 2+

Skin: Cool, dry, pallor

Musculoskeletal: Full ROM

Neuro: GCS of 8, not able to follow commands.

Laboratory/Imaging and Pertinent Initial Findings

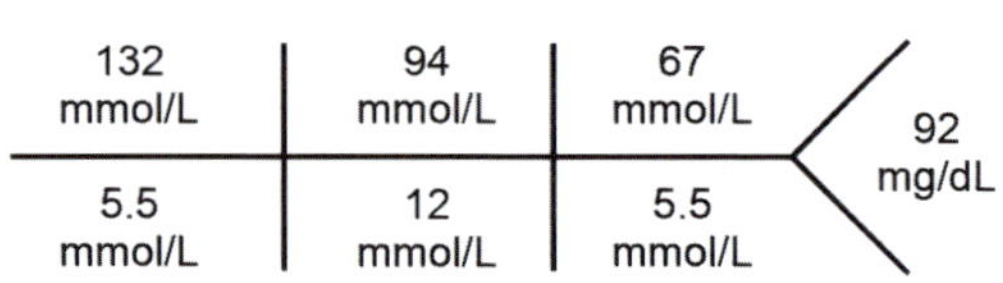

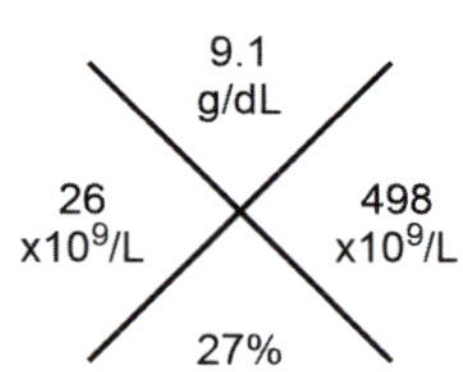

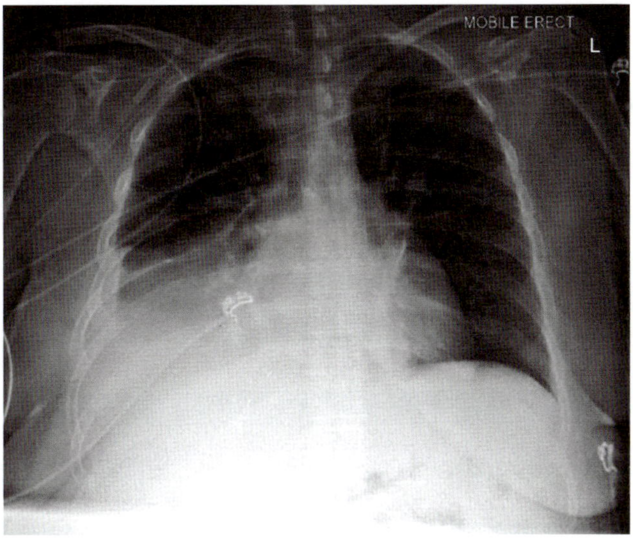

Fig. 10.1: Chest X-ray with right lobe pneumonia diagnosis

Arterial blood gas: pH 7.1, pCO_2 64, pO_2 62, Bicarb 13
Lactic acid: 10 mmol/L
Foley placed in the ER with no urine output
Capillary refill time >10 seconds
Chest XR with concern for right lower lobe pneumonia.

DEFINING SHOCK

- Shock is defined as a circulatory failure with inadequate tissue perfusion resulting in tissue hypoxia.
- Diagnosis of shock is usually based on multiple factors which include clinical, hemodynamic, and lab abnormalities.
  - Clinical signs typically include but are not limited to altered mental status, cold/clammy skin, and a drop in urine output.
  - Hemodynamic abnormalities with hypotension and tachycardia are usually patient-specific. Current guidelines recommend aiming for a mean arterial pressure (MAP) of 65, anything less than this is considered hypotension. Patients with baseline hypertensive might benefit from a higher MAP for adequate tissue perfusion.
  - Lab abnormalities typically reveal elevated lactic acid which can be a surrogate marker for abnormal tissue oxygenation.

INITIAL SHOCK ASSESSMENT

Basic Monitoring

Blood Pressure

- Noninvasive BP (NIBP) monitoring is the initial step in the assessment of a patient in the ICU in shock.
- Studies looking at the utility of NIBP *vs* arterial line are limited and have failed to show a benefit of arterial line over NIBP measurements. (Lakhal, Macq et al. 2012) (Gershengorn, Wunsch et al. 2014)

- Arterial lines have utility in patients who require frequent arterial blood gas collections or who need a closer evaluation of fluid responsiveness.
- Current recommendations are to maintain mean arterial blood pressure >65 with studies showing worse outcomes in patients with sustained MAP <65. (Maheshwari, Nathanson et al. 2018), (Khanna, Maheshwari et al. 2019).

Respiration

- Respiratory rate can be used to assess if the patient is in distress, tachypnea and bradypnea might be signs of impending respiratory collapse.
- Standard Pulse ox (SaO_2) is the most commonly used non-invasive method to measure oxygenation. It is used to measure transcutaneous oxygen saturation of hemoglobin in arterial blood. Pulse Ox does have certain limitations based on race and ethnicity (Wong, Charpignon et al. 2021).
- SaO_2 via arterial blood gas (ABG) is another method to assess oxygenation in patients with concerns for hypoxemia. Studies suggest that SaO_2 greater than 92% can be safely used to rule out hypoxia as defined by SaO_2 <90 %. (Gershengorn, Wunsch et al. 2014).

Cardiac Monitoring

- Continuous EKG
  - Can be used to evaluate ongoing arrhythmia.

Initial Labs/Physical Exam/Imagining

- Complete blood count
- Basic metabolic panel
- Lactate
  - Is a surrogate marker for tissue hypoxia/hypoperfusion
  - Serum lactate >2 mmol/L (18 mg/dL) has been used as a marker for circulatory abnormalities. (Singer, Deutschman et al. 2016), (Sauer, Gómez et al. 2021)
- ABG (especially if concerns for hypoxic/hypercapnic respiratory failure).
- Mixed venous oxygenation (SvO_2)
  - Measures oxygen saturation from mixed venous blood.
  - Used as a marker of oxygen extraction in the body.
  - Normal SvO_2 ranges from 65–70%
  - High SvO_2 is seen in states of increase O_2 delivery or decrease demand
    - Distributive shock.
  - Low SvO_2 is seen in states of low O_2 delivery
    - Hemorrhagic shock, cardiogenic shock, obstructive shock.
  - Accurate measurement requires placement of pulmonary artery catheter. Studies comparing correlation between SvO_2 and $ScvO_2$ (Central venous saturation) have shown poor reliability with $SvO_2 > ScvO_2$ (van Beest, van Ingen et al. 2010)
- Capillary refill time
  - Refill time > 3 sec considered abnormal
  - CRP is easy to assess and shows rapid improvement with resuscitation
  - But resuscitation aimed at targeting CRP *vs* lactic did not show improved mortality. (Hernández, Ospina-Tascón et al. 2019)

- Blood and urine cultures if concerns for septic shock
- Appropriate imagining study pertinent to patients' history.

Point of Care Ultrasound

- Point of care ultrasound if available can be used rapidly to assess:
  - Pump: Heart
    - Looking at the pericardial sac, heart chambers contractility, and valves.
  - Pipe: Aorta
    - Assessment of dissection, aneurysms
  - Tank: IVC and venous system
    - IVC distention, B lines, pleural fluid.
    - Obstruction in the tank, for example, in a pneumothorax.

Initial Approach

Antibiotics

- Early administration of antibiotics in patients with sepsis has the strongest evidence behind it with the current society of critical care guidelines recommending administration within one hour of recognition of sepsis or septic shock.
- Initial antibiotics should be broad spectrum and account for patient's prior culture data if available along with local resistance rates for common infectious pathogens.
- Antibiotics can be narrowed down after further culture data becomes available.

Oxygenation

- Administration of oxygen should start immediately to increase oxygen delivery.
- Oxygen delivery is one of the pivotal aspects of the management of shock. Oxygen content in the blood (CaO_2) is the amount of oxygen bound to hemoglobin plus oxygen devolved in blood, with the equation as noted below.
  - CaO_2 (mL O_2/dL) = (1.34 × hemoglobin concentration × SaO_2) + (0.0031 × PaO_2)
  - SaO_2 is the oxygen saturation and PaO_2 is the partial pressure of O_2 from the ABG.
  - Oxygen delivery to the microcirculation is defined as DO_2 (mL/min) = Q × CaO_2, where Q is the cardiac output.
- Initial administration of supplemental oxygen with non-invasive methods like nasal cannula and high flow nasal cannula should be initiated on initial presentation unless the patient is unable to protect their airway or is in severe respiratory distress.
- Some of the studies have suggested that early intubation in patients with septic shock with hypoxia might have better outcomes. (Yang, Shen et al. 2021)
- The use of a high-flow nasal cannula has been evaluated as an alternative for patients with hypoxia associated with shock. (Jhou, Chen et al. 2020)

Fluid Administration

- Fluid therapy is aimed at improving blood flow along with increased cardiac output.
- Current surviving sepsis guidelines recommend the administration of at least 30 mg/kg of IV crystalloid as part of initial resuscitation.
- The central dogma is changing from the administration of a set bolus of IVF to patients with shock to an assessment of fluid responsiveness periodically before additional fluid administration.

- The gold standard to assess hemodynamics and fluid responsiveness has been the use of pulmonary artery catheters but the use of noninvasive and bedside assessment strategies has been gaining popularity and are increasingly used in the setting of shock.
  - Some of the common non-invasive ways to measure fluid responsiveness are:
    - **Static**
      - Central Venous Pressure (CVP)
        - Has poor data behind it and does not generally correlate well with dynamic testing.
      - IVC variability
        - IVC can be used to estimate right atrium pressures in non-ventilated patients by looking at its diameter and collapsibility.
          - A patient with a diameter of <21 mm with collapsibility of >50% during inspiration likely has normal RA pressures between 0–5 mmHg.
          - A patient with a diameter >21 mm with <50% collapsibility during inspiration likely has elevated RA pressures (greater than 10 mmHg).
        - A change in IVC diameter with the respiration of 12–18% has been associated with fluid responsiveness in mechanically ventilated patients but the sensitivity and specificity in the systemic review have been poor.
    - **Dynamic**
      - Passive leg raising
        - Transiently increase venous return by elevating patients' legs at 45 degrees.
        - Responsiveness is considered to be an improvement in cardiac output of greater than 10% within 60–90 seconds.
      - Pulse pressure variation (PPV)
        - Patients need to be mechanically ventilated, with no spontaneous breaths with tidal volume >8 cc/kg of ideal body weight, and have no underlying arrhythmia. (Heenen, De Backer et al. 2006)
        - Normal pulse pressure variation is defined as 13%, patients that have pulse pressure variation less than 13% are not considered to be fluid responsive. (Michard, Boussat et al. 2000), (Yang and Du 2014)
      - Stroke volume variation
        - Have the same limitations as a pulse pressure variation
        - A value greater than 15% after receiving a 500 cc bolus of fluids.
      - Point of care ultrasound with velocity time integral (VTI)
        - VTI is the measurement of blood flow during systole through the left ventricular outflow tract (LVOT)
        - The normal VTI range is 18–22 and generally values below this are suggestive of cardiac depression.
        - An increase in the VTI in a patient with a fixed LVOT is considered to be fluid-responsive.
        - VTI is evaluated using five-chamber apical and parasternal views.
        - An average of 3 measurements in patients in sinus rhythms (of 5 in patients with atrial fibrillation) are evaluated.
        - An increase of 10% is consistent with fluid responsiveness.
- Continued maintenance of IVF in patients who presented in shock is of limited value. (Malbrain, Van Regenmortel et al. 2018)

- The choice of IVF fluids has changed over the years, most recent data suggest the use of balanced crystalloids with LR. (Semler, Self et al. 2018) over the use of normal saline and albumin.

Vasopressors

- In cases of severe hypotension with ongoing end-organ dysfunction despite IVF initiation vasopressors are indicated to prevent further hemodynamic instability. (Vincent and De Backer 2013)
- Adrenergic agonists have a rapid onset along with a short half-life which makes them ideal agents to be used in patients with ongoing shock.
  - Beta receptor stimulants increase blood flow but also increase myocardial oxygen demand with the risk of worsening myocardial ischemia.
  - Alpha receptor stimulants increase vascular tone along with BP but also decrease cardiac output.
  - Agents which have a favorable profile typically have a combination of both alpha and beta activity.
    - Norepinephrine is generally regarded as a first-line vasopressor that exerts most of its activity through alpha receptors with some beta stimulation. (Permpikul, Tongyoo et al. 2019)
    - Epinephrine has strong beta activity but some alpha activity at higher doses. Epinephrine can increase the risk of arrhythmia and decrease splanchnic blood flow. It is currently regarded as a third-line vasopressor. (Annane, Vignon et al. 2007, Levy, Perez et al. 2011)
    - Dopamine which has beta activity at lower doses with alpha activity at higher doses was initially used as a choice of vasopressor given its theoretical reno-protective profile. Multiple recent RCTs have shown no overall improvement in outcomes and was associated with increased risk for arrhythmia and death. (De Backer, Biston et al. 2010, De Backer, Aldecoa et al. 2012)
  - Other vasopressors
    - Vasopressin
      - Is responsible for vasoconstriction by activation of V1a receptor on the vascular smooth muscles.
      - Per the surviving sepsis guidelines vasopressin is regarded as a second-line vasopressor after norepinephrine. (Evans, Rhodes et al. 2021)
      - Vasopressin alone has not shown to have improved. (Russell, Walley et al. 2008)
    - Angiotensin II
      - Has been shown to improve outcomes in patients with vasodilatory shock who were already on other vasopressors. (Khanna, English et al. 2017)
      - Studies on its use are currently ongoing.
    - Steroids
      - Have mixed data on its efficacy in clinical trials. (Annane, Renault et al. 2018, Venkatesh, Finfer et al. 2018)
      - More studies are ongoing.
    - Methylene blue and hydroxocobalamin
      - No RCT, data supporting its use is mainly case report derived.

CLASSIFICATIONS OF SHOCK AND DISTINGUISHING FEATURES

- Shock is unique in that it is a diagnosis with multiple etiologies. Shock can be divided into 4 main categories: Distributive, cardiogenic, obstructive, and hypovolemic. These four categories vary in their etiologies, presentation, course, and treatment. To treat shock, you must diagnose correctly. In this section, we explore the hemodynamic variation between classes of shock and discuss causes and interventions.
- Tools to distinguish shock
  - Distinguishing types of shock typically require an understanding of cardiac output, systemic vascular resistance, central venous pressure, mean arterial pressure, and mixed venous oxygen saturation.
  - Cardiac output allows for calculation of systemic vascular resistance which is one of the few assessments that has been proven to be shock class specific. (Vahdatpour, C)
    - SVR is calculated by this formula SVR = ((MAP–CVP)/CO) × 80
    - MAP = Mean arterial pressure
    - CO = Cardiac output
    - CVP = Central venous pressure
    - Normal SVR is 800–1600
    - SVR less than 800 is associated with distributive shock
    - SVR above 1600 is associated with cardiogenic shock
  - The most widely accepted method for calculating cardiac output is via thermodilution in a PA catheter. Other less supported methods include using Fick's formula and external monitors to calculate CO.
  - Pulmonary capillary wedge pressure (PCWP) is another measure used to differentiate other forms of shock
    - This is an indirect measure of left ventricular end-diastolic function.
- Central venous pressure is measured by a catheter within the right atria.

Distributive Shock

- Distributive shock is defined as a state of relative hypovolemia due to immune-mediated dysfunction of the vascular endothelial system. There are three main types of distributive shock: Septic, anaphylactic, and neurogenic.
- The three main subtypes of distributive shock are all characterized by similar hemodynamic parameters:
  - Decreased SVR, increased CO, increased SvO_2, variable PCWP, and CVP
  - Further subtypes are distinguished based on etiology and physical exam findings which are detailed below.

Septic Shock

- Septic shock is the most extreme version of sepsis caused by dysregulation of the immune system leading to systemic circulatory failure and end-organ damage to hypoperfusion.
- Septic shock is distinct from other distributive shocks in that the immune system becomes dysregulated in response to an infection. The immune system triggers a cascade that relaxes the blood vessels, reducing tone and slowing forward blood flow. (Elbers, P., W., et. al. 2006)

- Septic shock is by far the most common type of shock. In a large study of shock cases over 60% are attributed to sepsis (De Backer). In addition to being the most common form of shock it is also the deadliest. Septic shock, kills one in four (Angus., D, Linde-Zwirble., et al. 2001) (Fleischmann-Struzek, C Mellhammar, et. al 2020)
- Septic shock can occur in anyone, but certain individuals and conditions are predisposed to higher rates of sepsis and are found to have worse outcomes.
- Individuals at higher risk of septic shock are the elderly, neonates, patients with diabetes, and immunocompromised and cirrhotic patients. When encountering a patient with any of these risk factors, an infectious etiology of shock should rise on your differential. (Singer, Deutschman et al. 2016)
- **Distinguishing features**
  - Extremes in temperature are associated with septic shock. Fever is a hallmark of sepsis and points toward an infective process of shock. Hypothermia can also be an indicative of severe septic shock.
  - Other physical exam findings include tachycardia, skin rash, warm extremities, and altered mental status. Patients with septic shock are warm and often diaphoretic.
  - As discussed above elevated SvO_2 and decreased systemic vascular resistance, tachycardia, and increased CO resistance are specific to distributive shock.
  - Important physical exam findings that indicate septic versus other forms of shock are the clinical suspicion for a source of infection.
  - Clinical findings indicative of infection:
    - Concern for source: Such as skin infections (cellulitis), presence of wounds, respiratory illness (PNA), urinary system, or GI tract infections. Typical symptoms of infection, even if mild, can be a clue that there is an infectious component causing shock.
    - Elevated leukocytosis or leukopenia white count above 10> or less than 5< are consistent with an infective nature of the shock.
    - Elevated inflammatory markers; CRP, ESR, and if concern for respiratory involvement elevated procalcitonin. CRP is the most sensitive of the inflammatory markers but the least specific.
    - Fluid responsiveness distinguishes septic shock from other forms. Patients with sepsis will have an increase in MAP and a decrease in lactic acid with appropriate fluid replacement per the current guidelines published in the meta-analysis Surviving Sepsis Campaign International Guidelines (Evans, Rhodes et al. 2021).

Anaphylactic

- An anaphylactic shock is an immune-mediated form of distributive shock. However, this is due to a severe systemic hypersensitive reaction.
- The presentation of anaphylactic shock is acute in onset and defined by possible life-threatening airway compromise and a decrease in circulation due to a lack of tone within blood vessels.
- This response is defined by overstimulation of IgE and activation of mast cells (Reber). This type of shock is acute and life-threatening. Treatment requires airway support and rapid administration of epinephrine. (Korhonen, H., Fisslthaler, B., 2009)
- **Distinguishing features**
  - Laryngeal edema, erythema, total body edema, tachypnea, tachycardia.

Neurogenic

- Neurogenic shock is caused by injury to the spinal cord. Most common in higher spinal cord injuries.
- Typically cause is due to loss of sympathetic tone and unopposed parasympathetic response. Generally neurogenic shock is associated with trauma to the spine but other causes including Guillain-Barré syndrome, autonomic nervous system toxins, and transverse myelitis have been associated with this form of shock. (Taylor, M. P., Wrenn, P., et al.)
- **Distinguishing features**
  - This type of shock is characterized by hypotension, bradyarrhythmia, and temperature dysregulation.
  - History of recent trauma to the spinal cord, exposure to neurogenic toxins, or history of demyelinating disease.

Cardiogenic Shock

- Cardiogenic shock (CS) is a hemodynamically complex and multifactorial syndrome characterized by systemic hypoperfusion and tissue hypoxia, generally due to primary myocardial insult or dysfunction (Baran et al., 2019).
- The etiology of the primary cardiac injury may be related to the pericardium, myocardium, valves, or conduction system (van Diepen et al., 2017).
- The hemodynamic criteria that are used to define cardiogenic shock were outlined in a review by Abraham et. al and include two main items: Hypotension (generally defined as systolic blood pressure < 90 for > 30 minutes and/or use of vasoactive/inotropic medications or MCS to maintain SBP > 90), and hypoperfusion (i.e. serum lactic acid > 2 mmol/L, acute kidney injury, acute liver injury, altered mental status) (Abraham et al., 2021).
- In 2019, the Society for Cardiovascular Angiography and Interventions (SCAI) proposed a new classification schema that outlines simple and clinically based definitions for the stages of cardiogenic shock as outlined below (Baran et al., 2019).
  - SCAI-A ("at risk"): Patient has risk factors for a cardiogenic shock with no signs or symptoms.
  - SCAI-B ("beginning"): Patient has evidence of relative hypotension or tachycardia WITHOUT hypoperfusion.
  - SCAI-C ("classic"): Patient WITH evidence of hypoperfusion requiring inotrope, pressor, or MCS.
  - SCAI-D ("deteriorating"): Patient failed to respond to initial interventions, clinically worsening with the above support.
  - SCAI-E ("extremis"): Patient has refractory cardiogenic shock while supported by multiple interventions, is highly unstable, often experiencing cardiovascular collapse.
- **Etiology of cardiogenic shock**
  - Broadly speaking, the majority of CS patients fall into the AMI or HF cardiogenic shock phenotypes, which have distinct pathophysiologic processes that drive the clinical syndrome. It is important to distinguish whether the cardiogenic shock is AMI versus HF phenotype as it has significant implications for management. (Baran)

- AMI CS is characterized by an abrupt reduction of contractility triggered by primary myocardial ischemic insult (i.e. STEMI, NSTEMI). This ischemic insult is followed by hypotension, with hypoperfusion and congestion as later clinical findings.
- Conversely, the HF CS patient generally presents with acute decompensated heart failure with congestion as their presenting symptom, which ultimately leads to hypoperfusion and hypotension as later clinical findings.

• **Distinguishing features**
  - The generally accepted signs of tissue perfusion include tachycardia, pale cool, and clammy peripheries with prolonged capillary refill time, oliguria, and altered mental status (Shah et al., 2019).
  - Other findings may include S3 gallop on a cardiac exam, elevated jugular venous pulses, pulmonary rales, lower extremity edema, pulsatile liver, and abdominal ascites which could be signs of congestion.
  - The highest yield labs for the diagnosis of cardiogenic shock are elevated lactate and mixed venous saturation (SvO_2) of less than 65% (Shah et al., 2019)
  - Brain natriuretic peptic (BNP) labs are generally elevated in the setting of HF cardiogenic shock and are helpful for prognostication with these patients.
  - High-sensitivity troponin labs are useful to assess the severity of myocardial injury in cases such as AMI shock and fulminant myocarditis, and serial measurements are often followed in the setting of reperfusion to estimate the amount of cardiac necrosis (van Diepen et al., 2017).
  - A chest X-ray may be obtained to assess heart size and pulmonary congestion or identify other pathology such as acute aortic dissection or pneumothorax (van Diepen et al., 2017). An ECG is diagnostic for ACS patients, but can also provide useful information regarding alternate diagnoses such as electrolyte derangements, pulmonary embolism, acute myocarditis, or drug toxicity (van Diepen et al., 2017). Echocardiogram and right heart catheterization (RHC) are both extremely useful in assessing and managing these patients.
  - Echocardiographic data (whether transesophageal or transthoracic) may provide information regarding the chronicity of the disease, evidence of ischemic event (such as wall motion abnormalities), valvular pathology, volume status, characterize phenotype (left ventricular (LV), right ventricular (RV), or biventricular (Bi-V)), and identify specific pathology (i.e. tamponade, RV strain due to acute PE, elevated RVSP in the setting of underlying pulmonary hypertension).
  - **Special consideration for the management of patients in cardiogenic shock**
    - ❑ While the treatment of CS has advanced tremendously over the last several decades, mortality of CS remains high at 35–50%, without significant improvement despite these advances (van Diepen et al., 2017). There are many specific challenges for establishing evidenced-based care for these patients including the highly heterogeneous population and lack of prospective randomized control trials. The pinnacles of CS treatment are the optimization of preload, afterload, and contractility.
    - ❑ There is a myriad of therapies used for the treatment of cardiogenic shock patients which will not be discussed in detail at this time. Revascularization in select populations should be pursued if indicated.
    - ❑ Common medical therapies include vasodilators (particularly useful for CS patients with high systemic vascular resistance), diuretics, pulmonary vasodilators for select

patients, inotropic medications (dobutamine, milrinone), and vasoactive agents to maintain blood pressure. If patients fail to respond to the above therapies, further management may require mechanical circulatory support (MCS) including both univentricular or biventricular support.

Hypovolemic Shock

- Hypovolemic shock is characterized by a decrease in cardiac preload to the extent that large and small systemic circulations are affected.
- Causes of hypovolemic shock
  - Blood loss
    - Blood loss may be hemorrhagic or hemolysis in nature.
    - Acute hemorrhagic blood loss is primarily from traumatic injury. This is identified by the history of injury, large bruising, open wounds decreased blood counts on lab work with any of the above corroborating findings.
  - Fluid loss
    - Gastrointestinal losses
      - GI loss is the most common cause of fluid loss. This is due to the physiology of the GI tract.
      - 3–6 Liters of fluid are secreted by the GI tract daily and when functioning correctly are almost all reabsorbed. However, in presence of insult to GI tract, reabsorption is easily impaired causing a significant amount of fluid loss. (Taghavi, S., & Askari, R., 2019).
    - Renal losses
      - Loss of fluid through the renal system can occur when there is an injury to the kidney, inappropriate signally from the aldosterone pathway, imbalance of electrolytes, or from medication use/misuse.
      - Renal losses are less likely to lead to hypovolemic shock, but most common etiologies. (Taghavi, S., & Askari, R. (2019).
    - Diuretic use
      - Diuretics are prescribed in the treatment of heart failure and kidney disease to balance fluids and electrolytes in the setting of impaired ability to do so independently. When titrating these medications care must be taken not to cause over-diuresis and intravascular volume depletion.
- **Distinguishing features**
  - Unique findings will be overt volume loss from wound, injury, large hematoma, active GI loss in the form of diarrhea or vomiting, and increased urination.
  - A physical exam is consistent with cool extremities, delayed capillary refill, flat neck veins.
  - Lab work for hypovolemic shock will range from labs consistent with dehydration or severe anemia depending on the etiology.
  - Hemodynamic specifics: Increased SVR, increased CO, decreased CVP and PCWP. In addition, SvO_2 will be low.

Obstructive Shock

- Associated with an impediment in blood flow in the cardiovascular system. It is associated with any condition that impairs venous return, prevents diastolic filling, or elevated afterload.

- Most common causes are tension pneumothorax, pulmonary embolism, and cardiac tamponade.
- Cardiac tamponade
  - Restriction of cardiac filling with increased intrapericardial pressure.
  - Diagnosis by point-of-care ultrasound along with some physical exam findings of muffled heart sounds, JVD, and pulses paradoxus. With worsening effusions can also see electric alternans.
  - TTE findings of diastolic collapse of the RA (early sign) and collapse of the RV (specific).
- Pulmonary embolism
  - Sub-massive or massive PE can cause elevated pulmonary artery resistance which results in elevated RV afterload.
  - Diagnosis is made by CTA (computed tomography angiogram) or point-of-care ultrasound can also be used.
- Tension pneumothorax
  - Trapped air in the pleural space with ipsilateral lung collapse and mediastinal shift.
  - Diagnosis is made by physical exam, chest X-ray or point-of-care ultrasound.
- **Distinguishing features**
  - Obstructive shock is minimally responsive to fluids which is unique to obstructive shock.
  - Physical exam: Usually cool extremities, delayed capillary refill, increased JVP, variable heart and lung sounds.
  - Hemodynamically: Elevated CVP, increased PCWP, decreased cardiac output, and increased SVR.

BACK TO OUR PATIENT

Is this Patient in Shock?

- Yes, she meets the criteria of undifferentiated shock on arrival given her poor mental status, low urine output, prolonged capillary refill time along, and elevated lactate with low MAP.

What are the Initial Steps for this Patient?

- Differential for her shock includes: Septic (given her history of cough, physical exam findings, elevated white count), cardiogenic (history of heart failure with EF of 40–45%), hypovolemia (given her poor PO intake, significant diarrhea, and use of diuretics and SGLT2 inhibitors).
- Her mental status, pulse ox and ABG are all concerning for impending respiratory failure. She should be intubated, and a secure airway should be established.
- Septic shock should be high on the differential, and she should be started on broad-spectrum IV antibiotics which include coverage for gram-positive, gram-negative, and atypical organisms.
- Ideally these antibiotics would be started after appropriate cultures are collected but getting cultures should not delay the administration of antibiotics.
  - Blood/urine and tracheal cultures were collected.
  - She was started on Vancomycin and Piperacillin/Tazobactam.
- This patient is likely in septic shock but could also have a component of cardiogenic shock. Given low MAP and end-organ dysfunction, she should be given IVF. Following the current recommendations, we can start by giving her 30 mg/kg of LR over two hours.

Assessment of Workup of Shock

- After receiving IVF patient's BP remained stable at 94/43 with a MAP of 60 with an HR of 95 beats/min.
- POCUS was performed while she was in the ER which showed a hyperdynamic left ventricle.
- LV assessment was performed which showed a LVOT diameter of 2.1 cm with a VTI of 19 cm. This along with the patients' heart rate of 95 beats a minute gives us a cardiac output of 6.5 L/min.
- Based on the cardiac output of 6.5 L/min and a CVP of 14, patient's SVR was calculated at 566 (normal SVR is 700 to 1500).
- Low SVR, elevated HR and CO all indicate distributive shock (and likely septic in this patient with other findings of the infectious process)
- Given the MAP <65 and lactic acid of 11 despite receiving 30 mg/kg of IVF, passive leg raise was performed to assess fluid responsiveness.
  - Passive leg raise resulted in a CO increase of 9% not consistent with fluid responsiveness.
- Vasopressors were initiated to help maintain the MAP >65 and prevent further end-organ dysfunction.
  - Norepinephrine was started as the first line vasopressor with subsequent addition of vasopressin.
- Subsequent re-evaluation showed her MAP had improved to 70 along with a repeat lactic acid level of 8.
- Over the course of the next 24 hours her serum lactate improved to <2 and was able to successfully be weaned from vasopressin. She also has improvement in her urine output to now 20–30 cc/hr.
- Over the next couple of days, her vasopressors were stopped, her antibiotics narrowed based on her culture data of *Klebsiella pneumoniae* to ceftriaxone.

REFERENCES

1. Abraham, J., Blumer V, Burkhoff D, Sinha. S, & Kapur NK (2021). Heart Failure-Related Cardiogenic Shock: Pathophysiology, Evaluation and Management Considerations. Journal of Cardiac Failure, 27(10), 1126–1140.
2. Angus, D., et al. (2001). "Epidemiology of severe sepsis in the United States: Analysis of incidence, outcome, and associated costs of care." Critical Care Medicine: 29 (7): 1303–1310.
3. Annane, D., et al. (2007). "Norepinephrine plus dobutamine versus epinephrine alone for management of septic shock: a randomised trial." Lancet 370(9588): 676–684.
4. Annane, D., et al. (2018). "Hydrocortisone plus Fludrocortisone for Adults with Septic Shock." New England Journal of Medicine 378(9): 809–818.
5. Baran, D. A., Grines, C. L., Bailey, S., Burkhoff, D., Hall, S. A., Henry, T. D., Hollenberg, S. M., Kapur, N. K., O'Neill, W., Ornato, J. P., Stelling, K., Thiele, H., van Diepen, S., & Naidu, S. S. (2019). SCAI clinical expert consensus statement on the classification of cardiogenic shock. Catheterization and Cardiovascular Interventions, 94(1), 29–37.
6. Cannon, J. W. (2018). Hemorrhagic shock. "New England Journal of Medicine", 378(4), 370–379.
7. De Backer, D., et al. (2010). "Comparison of Dopamine and Norepinephrine in the Treatment of Shock." New England Journal of Medicine 362(9): 779–789.
8. De Backer, D., et al. (2012). "Dopamine versus norepinephrine in the treatment of septic shock: a meta-analysis*." Crit Care Med 40(3): 725–730.
9. Dhatariya, K. K. (2019). Defining and characterising diabetic ketoacidosis in adults. "Diabetes research and clinical practice," 155, 107797.

10. Diepen, S. v., Katz, J. N., Albert, N. M., Henry, T. D., Jacobs, A. K., Kapur, N. K., Kilic, A., Menon, V., Ohman, E. M., Sweitzer, N. K., Thiele, H., Washam, J. B., & Cohen, M. G. (2017). Contemporary Management of Cardiogenic Shock: A Scientific Statement From the American Heart Association. Circulation, 136(16), e232–e268.

11. Elbers, P.et al. (2006). "Bench-to-bedside review: Mechanisms of critical illness–classifying microcirculatory flow abnormalities in distributive shock." Critical care, 10(4), 1–8.

12. Evans, L., et al. (2021). "Surviving Sepsis Campaign: International Guidelines for Management of Sepsis and Septic Shock 2021." Critical Care Medicine 49(11): e1063–e1143.

13. Fincke, R., Hochman, J. S., Lowe, A. M., Menon, V., Slater, J. N., Webb, J. G., LeJemtel, T. H., & Cotter, G. (2004). Cardiac power is the strongest hemodynamic correlate of mortality in cardiogenic shock: A report from the SHOCK trial registry. Journal of the American College of Cardiology, 44(2), 340–348.

14. Fleischmann-Struzek, C., Mellhammar, L., Rose, N., Cassini, A., Rudd, K. E., Schlattmann, P,... & Reinhart, K. (2020). Incidence and mortality of hospital-and ICU-treated sepsis: results from an updated and expanded systematic review and meta-analysis. Intensive care medicine, 46(8), 1552–1562.

15. Gershengorn, H. B., et al. (2014). "Association Between Arterial Catheter Use and Hospital Mortality in Intensive Care Units." JAMA Internal Medicine 174(11): 1746–1754.

16. Heenen, S., et al. (2006). "How can the response to volume expansion in patients with spontaneous respiratory movements be predicted?" Crit Care 10(4): R102.

17. Hernández, G., et al. (2019). "Effect of a Resuscitation Strategy Targeting Peripheral Perfusion Status vs Serum Lactate Levels on 28-Day Mortality Among Patients With Septic Shock: The ANDROMEDA-SHOCK Randomized Clinical Trial." JAMA 321(7): 654–664.

18. Jhou, H.-J., et al. (2020). "High-flow nasal cannula therapy as apneic oxygenation during endotracheal intubation in critically ill patients in the intensive care unit: a systematic review and meta-analysis." Scientific Reports 10(1): 3541.

19. Kalra, S., Ranard, L. S., Memon, S., Rao, P., Garan, A. R., Masoumi, A., O'neill, W., Kapur, N. K., Karmpaliotis, D., Fried, J. A., & Burkhoff, D. (2021). Risk Prediction in Cardiogenic Shock: Current State of Knowledge, Challenges and Opportunities. Journal of Cardiac Failure, 27(10), 1099–1110.

20. Khanna, A. K., et al. (2019). "Association Between Mean Arterial Pressure and Acute Kidney Injury and a Composite of Myocardial Injury and Mortality in Postoperative Critically Ill Patients: A Retrospective Cohort Analysis." Crit Care Med 47(7): 910–917.

21. Khanna, A., et al. (2017). "Angiotensin II for the Treatment of Vasodilatory Shock." New England Journal of Medicine 377(5): 419–430.

22. Konstam, M. A., Kiernan, M. S., Bernstein, D., Bozkurt, B., Jacob, M., Kapur, N. K., Kociol, R. D., Lewis, E. F., Mehra, M. R., Pagani, F. D., Raval, A. N., & Ward, C. (2018). Evaluation and Management of Right-Sided Heart Failure. Circulation, 137(20), 578–622.

23. Korhonen, H., et al. (2009). Anaphylactic shock depends on endothelial Gq/G11. "Journal of Experimental Medicine," 206(2), 411–420.

24. Lakhal, K., et al. (2012). "Noninvasive monitoring of blood pressure in the critically ill: reliability according to the cuff site (arm, thigh, or ankle)." Crit Care Med 40(4): 1207–1213.

25. Levy, B., et al. (2011). "Comparison of norepinephrine-dobutamine to epinephrine for hemodynamics, lactate metabolism, and organ function variables in cardiogenic shock. A prospective, randomized pilot study." Crit Care Med 39(3): 450–455.

26. Lim, H. S., & Gustafsson, F. (2019). Pulmonary artery pulsatility index: physiological basis and clinical application. European Society of Cardiology (ESC), 32–28.

27. Maheshwari, K., et al. (2018). "The relationship between ICU hypotension and in-hospital mortality and morbidity in septic patients." Intensive Care Med 44(6): 857–867.

28. Malbrain, M. L. N. G., et al. (2018). "Principles of fluid management and stewardship in septic shock: it is time to consider the four Ds and the four phases of fluid therapy." Annals of Intensive Care 8(1): 66.

29. Michard, F., et al. (2000). "Relation between respiratory changes in arterial pulse pressure and fluid responsiveness in septic patients with acute circulatory failure." Am J Respir Crit Care Med 162(1): 134–138.

30. Morgan, B. (2018). Central Venous/Mixed Venous Oxygen Saturation. London Health Sciences Centre.

31. Nohria, A., Tsang, S. W., Fang, J. C., Lewis, E. F., Jarcho, J. A., Mudge, G. H., & Stevenson, L. W. (2003). Clinical assessment identifies hemodynamic profiles that predict outcomes in patients admitted with heart failure. Journal of the American College of Cardiology (JACC), 41(10), 1797–1804.
32. Orso D, Paoli I, Piani T, Cilenti FL, Cristiani L, Guglielmo N. Accuracy of Ultrasonographic Measurements of Inferior Vena Cava to Determine Fluid Responsiveness: A Systematic Review and Meta-Analysis. J Intensive Care Med. 2020
33. Permpikul, C., et al. (2019). "Early Use of Norepinephrine in Septic Shock Resuscitation (CENSER). A Randomized Trial." Am J Respir Crit Care Med 199(9): 1097–1105.
34. Russell, J. A., et al. (2008). "Vasopressin versus Norepinephrine Infusion in Patients with Septic Shock." New England Journal of Medicine 358(9): 877–887.
35. Sauer, C. M., et al. (2021). "Understanding critically ill sepsis patients with normal serum lactate levels: results from U.S. and European ICU cohorts." Scientific Reports 11(1): 20076.
36. Semler, M. W., et al. (2018). "Balanced Crystalloids versus Saline in Critically Ill Adults." New England Journal of Medicine 378(9): 829–839.
37. Shah, A. H., Puri, R., & Kalra, A. (2019). Management of cardiogenic shock complicating acute myocardial infarction: A review. Clinical Cardiology.
38. Singer, M., et al. (2016). "The Third International Consensus Definitions for Sepsis and Septic Shock (Sepsis-3)." JAMA 315(8): 801–810.
39. Taghavi, S., & Askari, R. (2019). Hypovolemic Shock.[Updated 2019 Jun 18]. StatPearls [Internet]. Treasure Island (FL): StatPearls Publishing.
40. Taylor, M. P.,et al. (2017). Presentation of neurogenic shock within the emergency department. "Emergency Medicine Journal, "34(3), 157–162.
41. Vahdatpour, C., Collins, D., & Goldberg, S. (2019). Cardiogenic shock. "Journal of the American Heart Association," 8(8), e011991.
42. van Beest, P. A., et al. (2010). "No agreement of mixed venous and central venous saturation in sepsis, independent of sepsis origin." Crit Care 14(6): R219.
43. Venkatesh, B., et al. (2018). "Adjunctive Glucocorticoid Therapy in Patients with Septic Shock." New England Journal of Medicine 378(9): 797–808.
44. Vincent, J.-L. and D. De Backer (2013). "Circulatory Shock." New England Journal of Medicine 369(18): 1726–1734.
45. Wong, A.-K. I., et al. (2021). "Analysis of Discrepancies Between Pulse Oximetry and Arterial Oxygen Saturation Measurements by Race and Ethnicity and Association With Organ Dysfunction and Mortality." JAMA Network Open 4(11): e2131674–e2131674.
46. Yang, T., et al. (2021). "Outcome after intubation for septic shock with respiratory distress and hemodynamic compromise: an observational study." BMC Anesthesiology 21(1): 253.
47. Yang, X. and B. Du (2014). "Does pulse pressure variation predict fluid responsiveness in critically ill patients? A systematic review and meta-analysis." Crit Care 18(6): 650.
48. Zern, E. K., Wang, D., Rambarat, P., Bernard, S., Paniagua, S. M., Liu, E. E., McNeill, J., Wang, J. K., Andrews, C. T., Pomerantsev, E. V., Picard, M. H., & Ho, J. E. (2022). Association of Pulmonary Artery Pulsatility Index With Adverse Cardiovascular Events Across a Hospital-Based Sample. Circulation, 15(2).

CHAPTER

11

Antibiotic Resistance in Intensive Care Units

Mudalige AD, Namalie KD

INTRODUCTION

Antibiotic resistance is defined as non-susceptibility of pathogens towards antibiotics. According to the European and USA Centre for Disease Prevention and Control, multidrug resistance is absent susceptibility to at least one antibiotic in three or more groups of antibiotics. Extensive drug resistance is defined as absent susceptibility to all but two or less groups of antibiotics. Pan drug resistance is when there is no susceptibility to any antibiotic.[1]

The prevalence of antibiotic resistance is rising globally and poses a major challenge in managing patients who are critically ill.[2] Intensive care units are unique locations with high density of antibiotic resistance as they have a vulnerable patient population who have undergone complicated surgical procedures and who are on immunosuppressive medications as well as broad spectrum antibiotics. Poor infrastructure with confined spaces and lack of commitment to infection control practices such as poor adherence to hand hygiene, inadequate decontamination, disinfection and sterilization of reusable equipment and unsatisfactory environmental cleaning coupled with staff inadequacy increase cross contamination and colonization with multidrug resistant microorganism.[3,4] The presence of invasive devices such as indwelling urinary catheters and central vascular access devices and numerous invasive procedures they undergo constantly threatens patient getting infected with multidrug resistant pathogens. With the emergence of antibiotic resistance and presence of critical illness, the risk of inadequate treatment can further escalate antibiotic resistance. Despite the belief of adequate dosing, critical illness, poor absorption, increase volume of distribution, reduce albumin, use of extracorporeal purification systems, altered pharmacokinetics, drug interactions, poor absorption and unpredictable pharmacodynamics due to the complex nature of this patient population there is serious doubt whether therapeutic levels of antibiotic concentrations are achieved in the patients' blood/tissues to counteract the bacteria. Unavailability of regular surveillance of drug concentrations in blood further aggravates this.

Among antibiotic resistant organisms, ESKAPE (*Enterococcus faecium, Staphylococcus aureus, Klebsiella pneumoniae, Acinetobacter baumannii, Pseudomonas aeruginosa, Enterobacter spp.*), multidrug resistant *Escherichia coli, Stenotrophomonas maltophil* and *Burkholderia cepacian* are important.

With high rates of antibiotic resistance, there is resultant higher rates of morbidity, mortality and health care cost directly due to antibiotics and indirectly due to increased length of stay.[5]

The following three case scenarios explain common multidrug resistant infections seen in ICUs in South East Asia.

CASE 1

A 40-year-old previously well patient is treated for pneumonia following a viral lower respiratory tract infection. Despite treatment with IV ceftriaxone 2 g daily, IV clarithromycin 500 mg 12 hourly and oseltamivir 75 mg 12 hourly, by day 5 he deteriorated and was intubated due to type 1 respiratory failure and transferred to intensive care unit (ICU). Antibiotics were escalated to IV meropnum 500 mg 12 hourly (eGFR-25 ml/kg/min) and IV levofloxacin 750 mg 48 hourly. He developed multiorgan failure and had to undergo continuous renal replacement therapy. By day 14 he was slowly recovering and was weaning on tracheostomy. On day 15, he developed new onset fever, with leukocytosis, rise in CRP, increased oxygen requirements and thick secretions from the tracheostomy tube. Blood, urine and respiratory samples for cultures and chest X-ray (Fig. 11.1) were repeated and a multidrug resistant organism *Acinetobactor baumannii* (Figs 11.2 and 11.3) which was only sensitive to colistin was isolated in the broncho-alveolar lavage culture. He was treated with colistin 2 million units 12 hourly for 8 days in combination with IV meropenem. By day 25 he was weaned from ventilator and decannulated from tracheostomy.

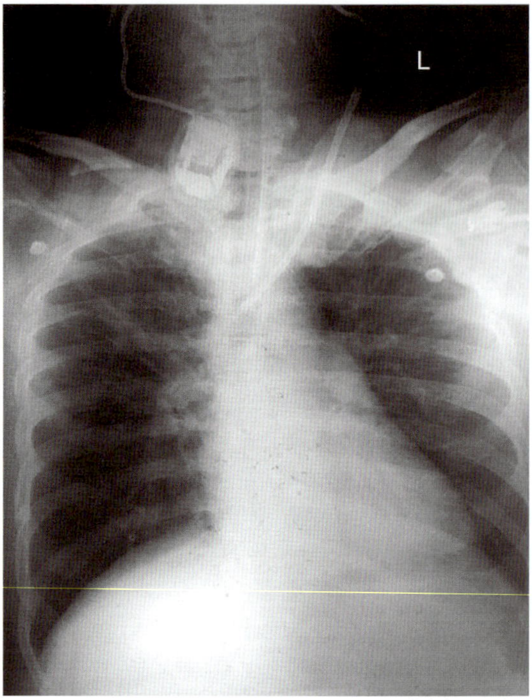

Fig. 11.1: Chest X-ray following deterioration of gas exchange showing new inflammatory shadows

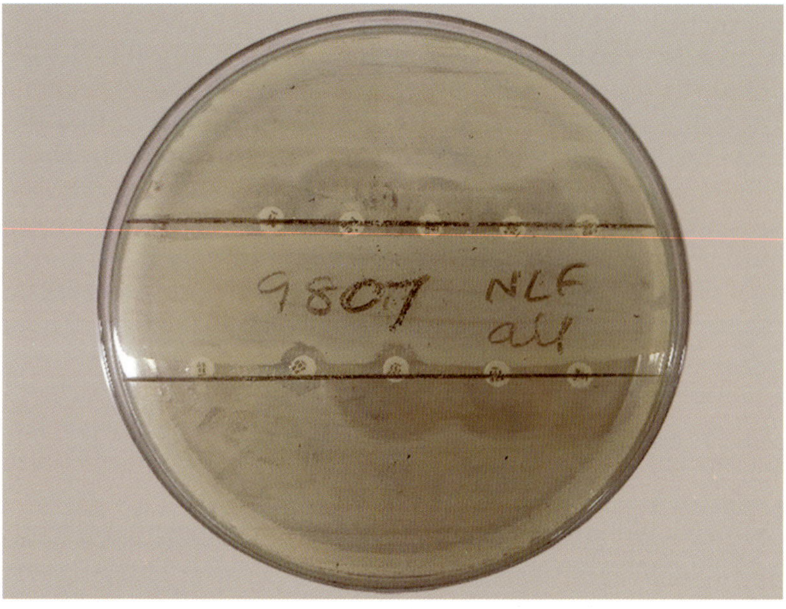

Fig. 11.2: Antibiotic sensitivity by John Stokes

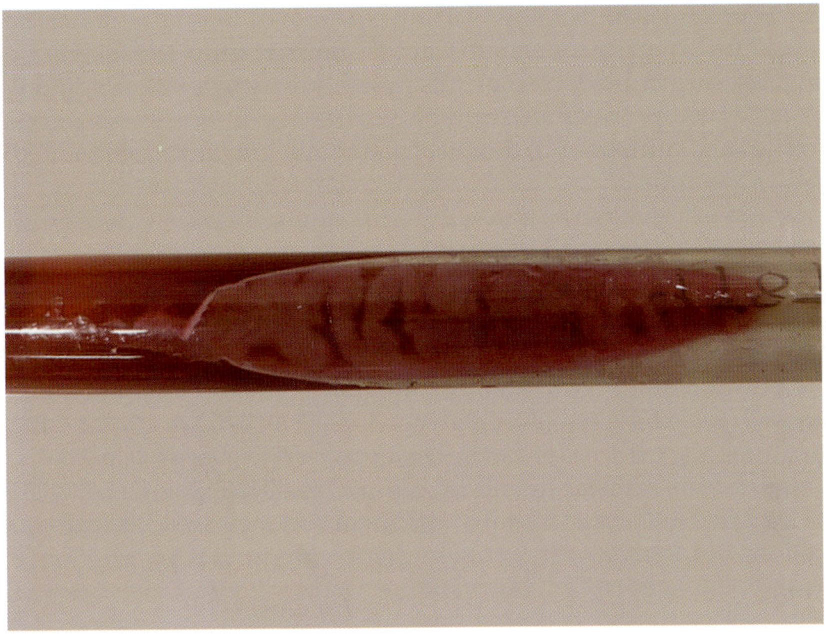

Fig. 11.3: Kigler iron agar slant from the isolate

Comparative Method

Acinetobacter spp are aerobic, gram negative, non-fermenting coccobacilli that are found in humid temperate climates. In hospital environment, the primary reservoirs of the organism are treatment areas, intensive care units, medical equipment, clinical staff and patients themselves. The propensity to cause nosocomial infections which are antibiotic resistant, has made it identified by the World Health Organization as a critical priority among organisms known to cause antibiotic resistance. The remarkable ability to acquire resistance to antibiotics is due to regulation of antibiotic transportation through bacterial membranes, alteration of the antibiotic target site and enzymatic modifications resulting in antibiotic neutralization.[6,7] It is known to cause ventilator associated pneumonia (VAP), surgical site infections (SSI), catheter associated urinary tract infections (CAUTI), blood stream infections as well as central line associated blood stream infections (CLABSI), wound infections and secondary meningitis. Increased length of hospital stay, ICU admission, exposure to invasive procedures, exposure to antibiotics (third generation cephalosporins, carbapenems, fluoroquinolones), use of steroids and host factors leading to severe immune compromise, predispose patients to acquire infections by *Acinetobacter spp*. *Acinetobacter spp* can lead to colonization without infection apart from clinical infection. It is important to differentiate the 2 conditions as the prior condition does not warrant treatment. The diagnosis is based on, along with suggestive clinical features a positive growth on the relevant specimen, for example, in a patient with fever, increased endotracheal secretions, deteriorating ventilator parameters and leukocytosis, a positive endotracheal culture or bronchoalveolar lavage culture. Treatment depends on the antibiotic sensitivity of the isolate.

Carbapenem resistant *Acinetobacter baunanii* (CRAB) infections are a frequent challenge in ICU settings. *Acinetobacter baumannii* has remarkable ability to acquire resistance to most other antibiotics expected to be active against wild-type when it is exposed to antibiotic pressure leaving a few remaining therapeutic options. The production of carbapenemases such as OXA carbapenemases, metallo-β-lactamases and additional serine carbapenemases,[8,9] further limits the utility of carbapenem agents. Sulbactam resistance is not completely understood but appears to be driven primarily via mutations targeting penicillin-binding proteins and β-lactamase production. Aminoglycoside modifying enzymes confer resistance to aminoglycosides and mutations in the chromosomally-encoded upregulated efflux pumps cause quinolone resistance.

Combination therapy with at least two active agents, whenever possible, is suggested for the treatment of moderate to severe CRAB infections. This is to be continued at least until clinical improvement is observed, because of the limited clinical data supporting any single antibiotic therapy. When the isolate is only sensitive to polymyxins as in this case, high dose polymyxins (polymyxin B or colistin) should be combined with high-dose, extended-infusion meropenem as a component of combination therapy for the treatment of moderate to severe CRAB infections. Tigecycline, which is a glycycline, also has efficacy for CRAB. Nebulized polymyxins or aminoglycosides also can be added although robust data to support this is not available. Finally, there is no clear "standard of care" antibiotic regimen for CRAB infections against which the effectiveness of various treatment regimen could be compared. Mortality of CRAB infections not treated with antibiotics appropriately is 70%.[10]

CASE 2

A 65-year-old male patient with type 2 diabetes on regular medication presented to ICU with acute chest pain and shortness of breath. He was diagnosed with COVID-19 by the SARS-CoV-2 lateral flow assay and confirmed by SARS-CoV-2 RTPCR. Chest X-ray (CXR) showed bilateral bronchopneumonia and admitted to ICU for respiratory support. C-reactive protein was rising from 130 to 157 and IV ceftriaxone was started suspecting secondary bacterial infection. Patient developed a non-ST-elevation myocardial infarction and went into cardiogenic shock needing ionotropic support. Patient's condition improved with standard COVID management and heparinization. His CXR was improved and was weaned off from respiratory support. Patient again developed spiking fevers, rising inflammatory markers and white cell count, and had to be started on inotropes. Septic screen was performed which included blood cultures from peripheral vein, central line and urine culture from the indwelling urinary catheter. Both central line and peripheral blood cultures grew *Klebsilla pneumoniae* with a difference in time to positivity more than 2 hours. Identification was by BD phoenix automated instrument and antibiotic sensitivities were performed by CLSI method. Central line associated blood stream infection was diagnosed and the central line was removed. The isolate was only sensitive to colistin and was classified by BD phoenix AST system expert rule, as a carbapenemase producer. The patient was treated with extended infusion high dose meropenem due to the non-availability of newer betalactam betalactamase combinations and colistin. Patient developed septic shock and organ failure and died on ICU day.[14]

Multidrug resistance gram negative bacteria, since their initial identification have progressed rapidly and have caused serious health consequences globally. Third generation cephalosporins were developed in the 1980s to overcome resistance against β lactamase bacteria. Within a few years of their use, extended spectrum β lactamase producing enterobacteria (ESBL) emerged with currently over 200 species identified imposing significant challengers to clinicians.[11] The prevalence of ESBL infections both in hospitals and in the community is rising.[12,13] Carbapenems are the antibiotics used to treat ESBL infections.[14,15] In the early 1990s carbapenem resistance was reported.[16] Since then, its rate of detection in hospitals as well as community is alarming.[17,18] The US Center for Disease Control defines carbapenem-resistant enterobacteria as isolates that are resistant to either imipenem, meropenem, ertapenem and doripenem. Carbapenem-resistant enterobacteria (CRE) impose major health concerns to the health care systems currently and is named one of the major threats to current human life by the World Health Organization.[17]

This heterogeneous group of pathogens with multiple potential mechanisms of resistance are broadly divided into those that are carbapenemase-producing and those that are not carbapenemase-producing. There are several carbapenemases produced by enterobacteria which include *Klebaiella pneumoniae* type carbapenemases (KPCs), New Delhi metallo-β lactamases (NDMs),[19] Verona integron-encoded metallo-β-lactamases (VIMs), imipenem hydrolyzing metallo-β-lactamases (IMPs) and oxacillinases (e.g. OXA-48-like).

Knowledge of whether a CRE clinical isolate is carbapenemase-producing and the specific carbapenemase produced is important in guiding treatment decisions especially with regard to newer antibiotics. The US Food and Drug Administration approved meropenem-vaborbactam, ceftazidime-avibactam, and imipenem-cilastatin relebactam are preferred treatment options for KPC-producing infections. Ceftazidime-avibactam in combination with aztreonam or cefiderocol as monotherapy, are preferred treatment options for NDM and other metallo-β-lactamase-producing infections while ceftazidime-avibactam is the preferred treatment for OXA-48-like-producing infections. Tigecycline and eravacycline are alternative options when β-lactam agents are either not active or unable to be tolerated. However, they are not recommended as monotherapy for the treatment of CRE bloodstream infections. Polymyxin B and colistin are effective but should be avoided for the treatment of infections caused by CRE whenever above agents are available. Carbapenem-resistant enterobacteria is commonly isolated in cases of VAP, CLABSI,[20] CAUTI and surgical site infections developed in ICU settings.

Prevention of CRE in ICU is a complex process. The use of broad spectrum antibiotics in the pre-ICU time period worsens the complexity. Screening for patients on admission to ICU (blood, sputum, faeces) through culture, rapid testing, isolation and treatment have been recommended with no definitive results. Hand hygiene, education of staff, vigilance and attempts to early detect infection, remain the cornerstones of control of CRE. Importance of practising bundle care for central line insertion and maintenance and conducting regular audits on practice of care bundles is emphasized through this case.

Of note is that SARS-CoV-2 pandemic has contributed to emergence of antibiotic resistance more than any other factor identified in the recent history.[1] The devastating global health situation led to fall in all aspects of prevention of antibiotic resistance and it is not unreasonable to state the aftermath of the calamity is yet to be seen.

CASE 3

A 16-year-old diagnosed patient with thalassaemia major presented to hospital with a history of fever, shortness of breath following 2 units of blood transfusion the previous day. Initially a transfusion reaction was suspected but the blood picture and antibody tests were not suggestive. The fever was persistent and there was hyperbilirubinaemia. She was investigated for the pyrexia and was treated with IV ceftriaxone 2 g daily for 2 days. Initial blood and urine cultures were negative. The initial ultrasound abdomen, chest X-ray and trans thoracic echocardiography were normal. There were high fever spikes which were persistent so antibiotics were changed to IV meropenem 1 g 8 hourly with IV teicoplanin 400 mg daily following three loading doses. As there was no response to broad spectrum antibiotics, transfusion associated infections due to repeated blood transfusions were suspected and blood for malaria parasite, serology for *Cytomegalovirus*, *Parvo* virus and *Epstein barr* virus were performed which were negative. Contrast enhanced CT scan of chest and abdomen were performed and CT abdomen revealed small liver abscesses which were not drainable. The blood and urine culture done on day 7 of ICU stay was positive for vancomycin resistant *enterococci* (VRE). The patient was suspected to have a CAUTI caused by VRE. She was isolated and treated with IV linezolid 600 mg 12 hourly and then fever responded. The supports were weaned off over a period of 10 days.

Enterococci are a group of gram positive, facultative, anaerobic cocci that are included in the genus streptococci present in the gastrointestinal system as commensal organisms. Of the many subtypes, *Entercoccus faecalis* accounts for most of the human infections (80–90%) while *Enterococcus facecium* (5–10%) is responsible for the rest.[21] Penicillin, and its derivatives are active against enterococcus *spp. Enterococci* have an extreme ability to develop both inherent and acquired resistance to antibiotics. Because of this, it is a common nosocomial organism in the hospital environment. *Enterococcus spp.* is inherently resistant to cephalosporins and frequent use of cephalosporin as empiric treatment has induced ampicillin resistance. As a result, the glycopeptides, vancomycin or teicoplanin has to be used in treatment regimens and use of glycopeptides leads to development of vancomycin resistance. For about 30 years, vancomycin was used to treat Enterococci infections resistant to other antibiotics until in late 1980s, the first report on vancomycin-resistant Enterococcus (VRE) was released from Europe. The realization that vancomycin was effective against *Clostridium difficile* and the rise in methicillin-resistant *Staphylococci* at this time, also contributed to an increased use of vancomycin. This led to the wide and rapid rate of spread of VRE around the globe.[22] The more so alarming fact would be this resistant pattern can be transmitted to other gram positive cocci for which the current standard treatment is vancomycin, a cautious reminder about how close we are to a catastrophic state of potentially untreatable killer bacteria with no effective antibiotics.[23]

VRE infections are the second most common health care associated infections and of the isolated *Enterococci* from CLABSI and CAUTI, 80% are VRE. Colonisation by VRE is also considerable and is quoted to be about one in ten infections. Colonization may be associated with higher risk of infection but treatment for colonization alone is not warranted. There are contradictory data on mortality with VRE infection which varies between no significant difference to 60–70%. CLABSI, CAUTI, surgical site infections, intra-abdominal abscesses and infections related to tubes, drains in abdomen following complex surgeries are common infections associated with VRE.

Risk factors for development of VRE are previous hospital admissions, duration of stay, previous use of antibiotics, especially 3rd generation cephalosporins and vancomycin and patient factors like immunocompromised states such as chronic kidney disease, malignancies and solid organ transplantation.[22] If not translocated from the internal milieu to cause infection, transmission is mainly through contaminated hands and equipment. The organism is believed to survive days to months on surfaces.

Diagnosis is based on clinical suspicion confirmed by culture of the culprit source. There are rapid molecular tests available for early diagnosis. The clinical significance of a positive culture during routine surveillance is not clear and does not warrant treatment at all times.

Treatment of enterococci infections as stated earlier requires a combination of drugs. Treatment of VRE, on the other hand, depends on the antibiotic sensitivity pattern. For UTI, ampicillin effective for susceptible isolates. Colonization alone warrants change of catheter. Antibiotics used in VRE are linezolid, daptomycin and tigecycline.[24]

Prevention of VRE infection is cost effective since treatment is difficult and time consuming. It is known that locations can be contaminated with VRE so cleaning of surfaces especially high touch surfaces and disinfection of equipment according to local guidelines is important. Surface surveillance helps in identifying these locations. Hand hygiene and staff education are of paramount importance. Colonizers and infected patients should be isolated in single rooms or kept in cohort isolation when single rooms are not available to prevent transmission to other patients. Use of barrier methods during attendance to patients is recommended. Since it takes a prolonged duration for clearance of the organism from the body, it is important to record this on discharge of the patient so the patient can be isolated during the subsequent admission to a hospital.

All 3 cases explain the challenges faced both by the treating party and the patient due to multidrug resistant infections in ICU. It reiterates the fact that all possible attempts to prevent these infections are warranted locally, nationally and globally. A more conservative approach in well-controlled conditions in treating patients with sepsis that limits early use of broad spectrum antibiotics until cultures are available, is a new concept that is emerging. To avoid under/overdosing, frequent review of antibiotic doses in each patient according to the level of illness, actual weight, renal and liver function and renal replacement therapy is essential. Monitoring therapeutic drug levels and dosing according to pharmacokinetic models will help to achieve effective minimal concentrations of antibiotics that were not achieved with traditional dosing. Early discontinuation of antibiotics after therapeutic goals achieved and de-escalation according to culture reports are a must in an effective antibiotic stewardship program. A change in perspective of antibiotic prescription towards more rational evidenced based approach is a much required need in the current context.

SUMMARY

Antibiotic resistance in ICU is a major hinderance to effective management of critically ill patients. A multitude of factors for decades have contributed to the development of serious resistance of bacteria to multiple groups of antibiotics. The condition leads to increased mortality, morbidity and cost in ICU but more alarmingly it will paralyse the medical system by allowing pan-resistant microbes to inhabit ICUs in the vey near future unless there is global acceptance of existence of the situation and planning of irreproachable combat is done without further delay.

REFERENCES

1. Na R C, Gijo D E and P Ruiz-Garbajosa. Antimicrobial resistance in ICUs: an update in the light of the COVID-19 pandemic. Curr Opin Crit Care 2020, 26:433–441.
2. Carleta J , Alib A B and Chalfinec A. Epidemiology and control of antibiotic resistance in the intensive care unit Current Opinion in Infectious Diseases 2004, 17:309–31632.
3. Tran G M, Ho-Le T P, Ha D T, Tran-Nguyen C H, Nguyen T S M, Pham TTN. Patterns of antimicrobial resistance in intensive care unit patients: a study in Vietnam, Curr Opin Crit Care 17:658–665T.
4. Duijna P J V, Dautzenberga M J D, Oostdijk E A N. Recent trends in antibiotic resistance in European ICUs Curr Opin Crit Care 2011; 17:658–665.
5. Kollef M H, Fraser V J. Antibiotic Resistance in the Intensive Care Unit. Ann Intern Med. 2001;134:298–314.
6. A.J. Varley, BSc MRCS FRCA, H. Williams, MB BCh FRCPath, S. Fletcher, FRCA FRCPE, Antibiotic resistance in the intensive care unit, Continuing Education in Anaesthesia Critical Care & Pain, Volume 9, Issue 4, August 2009, Pages 114–118.
7. Kyriakidis I, Vasileiou E, Pana ZD, Tragiannidis A. *Acinetobacter baumannii* Antibiotic Resistance Mechanisms. Pathogens. 2021; 10(3):373.

8. Wanger A, Chavez V, Huang R S P, Actor A W J, Dasgupta A. Chapter 7-Antibiotics, Antimicrobial Resistance, Antibiotic Susceptibility Testing, and Therapeutic Drug Monitoring for Selected Drugs. Microbiology and Molecular Diagnosis in Pathology,Elsevier, 2017, 119–153.
9. Timothy R. Walsh, Emerging carbapenemases: a global perspective, International Journal of Antimicrobial Agents 2010;36 (3): S8–S14.
10. Kim T, Lee EJ, Park SY, Yu SN, Lee YM et al. Natural prognosis of carbapenem-resistant *Acinetobacter baumannii* bacteremia in patients who did not receive appropriate antibiotic treatment: A retrospective multicenter study in Korea. Medicine (Baltimore). 2018 ;97(43):e12984.
11. Rawat D, Nair D. Extended-spectrum β-lactamases in Gram Negative Bacteria. J Glob Infect Dis. 2010 Sep;2(3):263–74.
12. Yousefipour M, Rasoulinejad M, Hadadi A, Esmailpour N, Abdollahi A et al. Bacteria Producing Extended Spectrum β-lactamases (ESBLs) in Hospitalized Patients: Prevalence, Antimicrobial Resistance Pattern and its Main Determinants. Iran J Pathol. 2019 Winter;14(1):61–67.
13. Xu Y, Gu B, Huang M, Liu M, Xu T et al. Epidemiology of carbapenem resistant Enterobacteriaceae (CRE) during 2000–2012 in Asia. Journal of Thoracic disease 2015; 7(3).
14. Paterson DL, Bonomo RA. Extended-spectrum beta-lactamases: a clinical update. Clin Microbiol Rev. 2005 Oct;18(4):657–86.
15. Pilmis B, Zahar J R. Ventilator-associated pneumonia related to ESBL-producing gram negative bacilli. Annals of translational medicine. Vol 6, No 21 (November 2018).
16. Joseph D. Lutgring, Carbapenem-resistant Enterobacteriaceae: An emerging bacterial threat, Seminars in Diagnostic Pathology, Volume 36, Issue 3, 2019, Pages 182–186.
17. Jones CD, Moore ZS, Sexton DJ, Anderson DJ. Rising rates of carbapenem-resistant enterobacteriaceae in community hospitals: a mixed-methods review of epidemiology and microbiology practices in a network of community hospitals in the southeastern United States. Infect Control Hosp Epidemiol. 2014 ;35(8):978–83.
18. Hu H, Mao J, Chen Y, Wang J, Zhang P et al. Clinical and Microbiological Characteristics of Community-Onset Carbapenem-Resistant Enterobacteriaceae Isolates. Infect Drug Resist. 2020 11;13:3131–3143.
19. Goodman K E, Simner P J, Tamma P D, Milstone A M. Infection control implications of heterogeneous resistance mechanisms in carbapenem-resistant Enterobacteriaceae (CRE) Expert Review of Anti-infective Therapy 2016:14(1):95–108.
20. Logan L K, Carbapenem-Resistant Enterobacteriaceae: An Emerging Problem in Children, Clinical Infectious Diseases, Volume 55, Issue 6, 15 September 2012, Pages 852–859.
21. Cetinkaya Y, Falk P, Mayhall CG. Vancomycin-resistant enterococci. Clin Microbiol Rev. 2000 ;13(4):686–707.
22. Rice L B. Emergence of Vancomycin-Resistant Enterococci Vol. Emerging Infectious Diseases 2001;7(2): 183.
23. Murray B E. Vancomycin-resistant enterococci. The American Journal of Medicine 1997;102(3): 284–293.
24. Levitus M, Rewane A, Perera TB. Vancomycin-Resistant Enterococci. [Updated 2022 Jul 18]. In: StatPearls [Internet]. Treasure Island (FL): StatPearls Publishing; 2022 Jan-. Available from: https://www.ncbi.nlm.nih.gov/books/NBK513233/
25. Brinka A J, Richards G. Best practice: antibiotic decision-making in ICUs. Curr Opin Crit Care 2020, 26:478–488.

CHAPTER

12

Invasive Fungal Infection in ICU

Veronica Lisseth Hernandez González, Maria Ortega Alaminos, Marcio Borges Sa

CASE PRESENTATION

A 65-year-old woman who came to the emergency department (ED) in January 2021 for 4 days of fever up to 38.6°C, asthenia, cough, whitish expectoration and increase in his usual dyspnea. She is a hypertensive patient with COPD and non-insulin-dependent diabetes mellitus. He has been using low doses of corticosteroids for months. In the ED, leukopenia with lymphopenia, elevated fibronogen and LDH, mild thrombopenia, very high CRP, normal procalcitonin. He had severe respiratory failure with no other organic dysfunctions. Optiflow is started in the ED. The patient remained in the ED for 6 hours, but due to deterioration the ICU was notified and it was decided to admit him urgently, proceeding to orotracheal incubation and initiation of invasive mechanical ventilation (IMV).

Blood cultures (negative), urine antigens (negative), bronchoaspirate after incubation (negative) and PCR for influenza (negative) and Covid-19, the latter being positive with a very low CT (which meant acute active infection), had already been taken in the emergency room. Chest X-ray showed bilateral and diffuse infiltrates. Treatment was started with corticosteroids, remdesevir and tociluzimab. Cefotaxime and levofloxacin were also prescribed for 5 days.

The patient presented a torpid evolution with development of severe ARDS in the first hours in ICU with alveolo-arterial gradients of 70, requiring prone decubitus. After the first 14 days of admission the patient had experienced a marked ventilatory improvement, so that the inspirate fraction of oxygen (IFO_2) could be lowered, and the patient was able to start weaning, but on the 18th day of admission to the ICU he presented new clinical deterioration. She presented with high fever, hypotension with shock requiring noradrenaline, new ventilatory deterioration requiring 100% IFO_2, acute renal failure. Regarding biomarkers, she presented intense leukocytes, with severe lymphopenia, very high CRP,

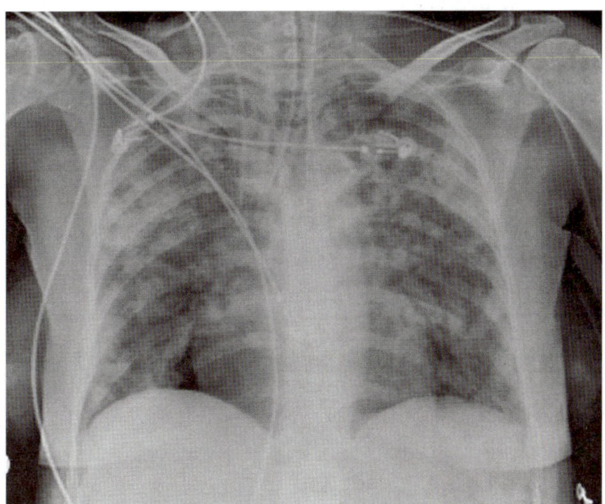

Fig. 12.1: Chest X-ray of the patient on the day of CAPA diagnosis

procalcitonin 0.9, creatinine 2.4, moderate thrombopenia. We proceeded to draw one and blood cultures, it was decided to perform fibrobronchoscopy and computerized topography. Broad-spectrum antibiotic treatment was started.

Finally, galactomonan was positive in the respiratory sample obtained by fibrobronchoscopy and an *Aspegillus fumigattus* was identified in the culture of the same.

Q. Should we always consider invasive pulmonary aspergillosis (IAP) in critically ill patients admitted to the ICU for Covid-19?

Ans: Yes, always. Invasive pulmonary aspergillosis is a diagnostic and therapeutic challenge in critically ill patients. The main reason is that we have different profiles of patients at risk, such as immunocompromised patients, on the one hand, and other types of patients such as COPD or influenza patients on the other.

An entity has even been defined as Covid-19 associate pulmonary aspergillosis (CAPA). It is a new patient profile, which usually combines traditional risk factors for IPA, such as severe lymphopenia, decreased IL-10, corticosteroid use, prolonged use of IMV, previous use of broad-spectrum antibiotics, hypertension, diabetes or COPD.

It is much less common for the patient to present with an acute co-infection of Covid-19 and an API. Most often, CAPA develops as a secondary complication, as a superinfection of patients with severe Covid-19 and who continue to be admitted to the ICU.

Therefore, in the case of a patient admitted to the ICU for Covid-19 who presents a complication and suspicion of superinfection, we should investigate the possibility of CAPA with all the microbiological tests available to us, and we should proceed to fibrobronchoscopy. Here the galacomannan obtained from the respiratory sample, mainly from bronchioalveolar lavage, has a much better yield than plasma. What does not seem to provide relevant information is the performance of a computerized topography. This is different from, for example, the study of IPA in neutropenic patients, where this imaging test is crucial for diagnosis and evolution.

Therefore, the suspicion of a CAPA is key to investigate a possible case in patients who present a superinfection in the evolution of a patient with Covid-19 complicated in the ICU.

Early and adequate initiation of antifungal treatment is crucial to reduce morbidity and mortality in patients with CAPA in the ICU. Both the initiation of empirical antifungal therapy in high-risk patients and targeted therapy after detection of aspergillus should be appropriate and adjusted according to the best PK/PD profile, appropriate dosage, with the lowest toxicity and drug–drug interactions. Triazoles are the antifungals of first choice, and voriconazole is the first choice and most experienced antifungal. But isavuconazole is also considered in recent CAPA guidelines to be the first choice, with obvious pharmacological advantages over voriconazole. If we cannot use them, liposomal amphotericin B is the alternative.

PRINCIPLES OF MANAGEMENT

Diagnosis

The diagnosis of IPA is made by combination of host factors, clinical, radiological features, and mycological evidence. The European Organization for Research and Treatment of Cancer/ Mycosis Study Group (EORT/MSG) established diagnostic criteria and risk factors for IPA for onco-hematological patients, however, in critically ill patients with CAPA said risk factors were present in only 12.5% of patients.[1,2]

Among the radiological criteria, the results are diverse, among them the most frequent are poorly defined and patchy condensations (63–76%), and secondly nodules (10–33%). Signs such as the "air crescent signs" or the inverted halo sign are only detected in 0.8–3.6% of cases.[3]

Laboratory procedures such as microscopy, culture, damage, and molecular techniques are used for microbiological diagnosis.[4]

The essential criteria for the diagnosis of IPA are the observation of hyphae in the microscopic analysis of a sample of sterile tissue, together with histological evidence of tissue invasion or isolation of *Aspergillus* in culture. However, depending on the type of sample, it can also indicate contamination of the sample or colonization of the bronchial tree,[4,5] so it must be noted that a positive culture from the upper respiratory tract, molecular detection (PCR) and /or antigen detection of *Aspergillus* species do not always indicate infection, rather these results will be detrimental as an indication to perform bronchoscopy and perform BAL especially in high-risk and immunocompromised patients in the ICU.[2,6,7]

Among biomarkers, galactomannan (GM) and B1, 3-D-glucan (BDG) remain the most widely used biomarkers. The determination by means of ELISA technique of GM fungal hardiness constitutes one of the diagnostic criteria of IPA according to the EORTC/MSG. However, in the non-neutropenic patient its diagnostic capacity decreases considerably.[8,9] It has been shown that even the determination of BDG in serum is superior to that of GM, but it is similar or inferior when compared to GM in BAL. Its main characteristic lies in its high negative predictive value (82–95%).[10,11]

There are currently a number of risk groups associated with IPA, including patients with COPD, *influenza virus* (IAPA), Covid-19, and immunodeficient patients such as an onco-hematology, mainly patients with prolonged and severe neutropenia and transplant recipients (mainly lung and bone marrow transplant recipients).

In patients with COPD, IPA should always be suspected, especially those who receive treatment with corticosteroids, present non-specific symptoms and radiological changes.[12,13] In patients with *influenza* infection, in addition to presenting IAPA (influenza-associated invasive pulmonary aspergillosis), it is noteworthy that the incidence of tracheobronchitis due to aspergillus is very high, up to 50%.[14]

On the other hand, in neutropenic patients, imaging tests such as chest computed tomography, detection of galactomannan in BAL, and bronchoscopy have greater diagnostic yield.

Currently an entity has even been defined as CAPA (Covid-19 associate pulmonary aspergillosis). This entity can present between the first and second week as a complication after Covid-19 infection with both clinical and radiological respiratory worsening. It is usually associated with risk factors such as the use of steroids, immunomodulators (such as tocilizumab), persistent lymphopenia, and duration of mechanical ventilation.[15]

It is proposed that CAPA be defined as possible, probable, or proven on the basis of sample validity and therefore diagnostic certainty.

An important difficulty in patients with Covid-19 is related to the findings in imaging tests such as radiographs and different CT patterns, especially in late stages. Atypical features of Covid-19 may suggest other diseases, such as lobar and segmental consolidation in the setting of bacterial pneumonia, or cavitation from necrotizing pneumonia.

It also highlights that the typical radiological characteristics of PAI (such as the halo sign) are not sufficient to define CAPA without mycological evidence, since in patients with Covid-19 this sign may also be present but is due to areas of local infarction. secondary to endotheliopathy thrombosis.[16]

Detection of GM in bronchoalveolar lavage does not prove tissue invasion, and the likelihood of infection is increased if circulating GM is detected. Unfortunately, the diagnostic yield of serum GM is low in CAPA as, at best, 20% of patients showed positive results and proven cases of CAPA with negative serum galactomannan have been reported.[17,18] In general, serum galactomannan has a reduced value to exclude CAPA.[19]

Finally, it can be said that for the diagnosis of CAPA, it is necessary to take into account the different clinical, radiological and mycological criteria, with culture and tissue microscopy showing the invasive growth of septate fungal hyphae in mainly sterile samples (biopsies or BAL) the diagnostic gold standard.

Treatment of Aspergillosis

Antifungal compounds used in the treatment of invasive aspergillosis.

Considerable expansion of antifungal pharmacological research and clinical development of various compounds has taken place in the last decade, resulting in new strategies and protocols.

Invasive pulmonary aspergillosis can progress to relentless and fatal pneumonia. In neutropenic patients this pneumonia can be characterized by a devastating hemorrhagic infarction or progressive necrotizing pneumonia.[1] If adequately treated, invasive pneumonia is further complicated by dissemination into the CNS or by extension to contiguous intrathoracic structures, including the great vessels and heart. Given the risk of extension and unfavorable evolution, early fungal treatment is essential for an adequate outcome. Early initiation of early and appropriate treatment is essential to achieve adequate outcomes in patients with a strong presumption of invasive aspergillosis, while an adequate diagnostic evaluation is performed. The decision to address invasive pulmonary aspergillosis with drug therapy is supported by several randomized controlled trials. Combination therapy is not recommended as primary treatment currently.[1,2,20] No randomized studies using combination treatments have been performed so far, and all available information comes from observational studies with different drug combinations and inclusion criteria, all with serious limitations, Therefore, there is no firm evidence at present for combination treatment of invasive aspergillosis. Future studies could answer so far unresolved questions.[20]

The duration of treatment depends on the location of the infection, the underlying disease and treatment response, and patient characteristics. Generally, it should be maintained for 12 weeks and until at least 2 weeks after the resolution of the patient's signs and symptoms, always taking into account the patient's possible immunosuppression and the risk of associated complications.[1,2,6,12,16,20,22] Surgical treatment is only indicated in cases of necrotizing sinusitis, necrotic skin lesions and pulmonary involvement with risk of hemoptysis.[22] In the case of chronic immunosuppression, continuation of antifungal therapy during immunosuppression appears to be associated with a more favorable outcome. There is a risk of recurrent infection of residual foci of infection that can be verified by imaging techniques and that would condition prolonged treatment.

In the following, we will describe the FDA-approved therapeutic strategies that will address the management of aspergillosis. They have both *in vivo* and *in vitro* activity and are licensed for the treatment of invasive aspergillosis: D-AMB and its lipid formulations, colloidal AMB suspensions, voriconazole, isavuconazole, itraconazole, posaconazole and caspofungin.

Voriconazole and D-AMB are the only ones licensed in the United States for the treatment of invasive aspergillosis. As a last resort, LFAB, itraconazole and caspofungin are approved for the treatment of invasive aspergillosis. Posaconazole is licensed for prophylaxis in myelodysplastic and neutropenic patients.

In the European Union, treatment with voriconazole is approved. As alternatives, isavuconazole and posaconazole are approved for the treatment of invasive aspergillosis in patients, but clinical experience is limited.

Recent API management and treatment guidelines in IAPA or CAPA suggest that both isavuconazole and voriconazole are the first indication antifungals, with liposomal amphotericin B (L-Amb) being the alternative in cases of resistance or side effects.[20,21] The use of posaconazole has a low experience. And the use of monotherapy with echinocandins is not recommended in general.[20,21]

Due to improved survival and favorable outcomes and favorable response to initial treatment with voriconazole, it is not recommended to initiate initial treatment with D-AMB (A-I). In most patients, oral or intravenously (IV) voriconazole is recommended for primary treatment (A-I). Treatment can be optimized orally at mg/kg or IV at an initial dose of mg/kg/12 h on the first day, thereafter at a dose of 4 mg/kg/12 h. For severe patients, always parenteral treatment is preferred. There is the possibility of using L-AMB as an alternative primary treatment, some drugs are: Posaconazole (B-II), Itraconazole (B-II), Caspofungin (B-II) or Micafungin (B-II).

For patients intolerant or resistant to voriconazole or others, azoles—an AMB formulation is an appropriate alternative. Historically, D-AMB has been used as a treatment for invasive aspergillosis.[1,2,6,12,20–22] But different studies have shown that L-AMB are equally effective for IPA and less nephrotoxic than D-AMB, they have also been considered for primary treatment against voriconazole, in those patients with a history of hepatic pathology, given the risk of hepatotoxicity of voriconazole. Treatment with itraconazole is not recommended in patients with contraindications or resistance to voriconazole, given the same mechanism of action or the possibility of resistance, bioavailability and risk of toxicity.[1,20–22]

But finally, Amphotericin B deoxycholate and itraconazole are no longer recommended as treatment against IPA. Currently the antifungal treatments used against API in ICU setting are: Triazols (voriconazole, isavuconazole and posaconazole), liposomal amphotericin B (L-Amp), and echinocandins (anidulafungin, caspofungin, micafungin).

Below, we describe the characteristics of the different groups of antifungal agents.

1. AMB (Amphotericin B)

AMB is a natural polyene macrolide antibiotic, it is not absorbed orally, its use is IV. After IV administration, it binds to proteins and is distributed in reticuloendothelial tissues (liver, bone marrow, lung, spleen) and kidney. It presents acute reaction in relation to administration, in addition to nephrotoxicity. Concentrations are reached after administration of 1 mg/kg IV, half-life of 24–48 h and terminal half-life >15 days. Nephrotoxicity is characterized by azotemia, ion loss and tubular acidosis.

Acute infusion-related reactions, chills, fever, nausea, arthralgias, headache and bronchospasm.

As we have previously commented, at present, if there are no economic problems restricting its use, L-AMB is the amphotericin of choice in severe patients with API.

2. Antifungal Triazoles

These are synthetic compounds that have a thiazole ring attached to the isobutyl nucleus or a carbon atom. They act on ergosterol biosynthesis by inhibiting the cytochrome P450-

dependent enzyme lanosterol, resulting in membrane disruption and cell death or growth inhibition, and also inhibit the cellular respiration chain.

The triazoles are the first option both empirical, pre-emptive as target antifungal therapy for API for critically ill patients and/or all risk group

Voriconazole

Voriconazole is presented IV or in tablet form, dissociates in plasma and follows its own disposition. It is eliminated mostly by the kidney, accumulation could generate nephrotoxicity and renal failure. The formulation presents good bioavailability. There are other adverse reactions such as hepatotoxicity, cutaneous exanthema and visual alterations.

The recommended dose is 6 mg/kg/12 h on the first day and 4 mg/kg/12 h thereafter.

This antifungal drug is the first choice in all groups of patients with API, but we have to take into account its potential problems: Eradicating dosage in critically ill patients, side effects, need for TDM, a large number of drug–drug interactions.[1,2,6,20,21]

Isavuconazole

Although with the recent inclusion of isavuconazole, it has also been incorporated as a first option in several reviews, expert documents or guidelines in patients with API, included in critically ill patients.[2,12,14,20,21] In comparison with voriconazole, isavuconazole has similar clinical efficacy but a clear PK/PD advantages, lower toxicity (e.g. neuro or hepatotoxicity) or incidence of drug interactions and no need for TDM. And the risk of QT prolongation with the potential risk of severe ventricular arrhythmias is minimal or non-existent with isavuconazole.

In particular, VRC was the antifungal of choice since it is the most studied so far. But at present, both voriconazole and isavuconazole should be considered drugs of choice for primary treatment of API in a COPD, influenza, Covid-19, hematological, neutropenics and HSCT patients considered as AI level of evidence.[2,5–7,12,14,16,20,21]

Itraconazole

It is a highly lipophilic compound of high molecular weight, its absorption increases with acid pH and lipid-rich diet. It is metabolized in the liver and excreted in bile and urine. The main adverse reactions are: Nausea and vomiting, increased triglycerides, hepatic failure and hypocalcemia, as well as cardiotoxicity.

The recommended dose is 2.5 mg/kg/12 h and orally 400 mg/day.

In daily clinical practice it is not an acceptable alternative in API in critically ill patients as it does not provide any advantage over voriconazole or isavuconazole and has more disadvantages, dosing problems and side effects.[20]

Posaconazole

It has a similar structure to itraconazole but only its oral formulation has been studied. It has two pharmacokinetics: Linear and saturable. It is mainly metabolized in the liver.

The dosage of the oral suspension is 200 mg 3 times a day as prophylaxis and 800 mg administered 2 or 4 times a day in treatment.

With the experience of voriconazole and the potential advantages of isavuconazole, posaconazole is a much less used and indicated alternative for the treatment of API in critically ill patients.[20,21]

3. Echinocandins (Caspofungin, Micafungin and Anidulafungin)

Echinocandins are currently only available via IV. They show a bioavailability proportional to the dose administered, with a half-life of 10–15 h, allowing a daily dose, which leads to easier administration. They show strong binding to proteins and their elimination is mainly through urine and feces, with hepatic metabolism in most cases.

Caspofungin is the most commonly used and is indicated in cases of probable or proven invasive aspergillosis, resistant or intolerant to first choice treatments. Caspofungin is administered 70 mg/day on the first day, followed by 50 mg/day.[2,6]

Micafungin and anidulafungin have activity against *Aspergillus spp* but are not approved or indicated and optimal doses have not been established.[20]

And finally, the echinocandins still play a less relevant role compared to triazoles or L-Amp. And there appears to be no difference between the three in efficacy against API. The option of monotherapy with echinocandins against API in critically ill patients continues to have low evidence and is generally considered as combination therapy.[2,6,12,20]

In short, IPA is a potentially serious entity, so greater emphasis is given to its treatment.[22]

FINAL CONSIDERATIONS

New patient profiles (such as Covid-19 patients) and risks factors have been emerging in recent years, which is why diagnostic and therapeutic individualization are key to improving the prognosis of these critical patients with API.

We need to make an active effort for early diagnosis of suspected cases of possible IPA in the ICU setting. Early CT, bronchoscopy, histological and microbiological tests are key for the diagnosis of API as well as other infectious or non-infectious etiologies.

Antifungal treatment in immunocompromised critically ill patients must have 3 main features: High efficacy, low interaction with other treatments and minimum adverse events.

REFERENCES

1. Koehler P, Bassetti M, Chakrabarti A, Chen SCA, Colombo AL, Hoenigl M, et al. Defining and managing COVID-19-associated pulmonary aspergillosis: the 2020 ECMM/ISHAM consensus criteria for research and clinical guidance. Lancet Infect Dis. 2021;21:e149–62.
2. Verweij PE, Brüggemann RJM, Azoulay E, Bassetti M, Blot S, Buil JB, et al. Taskforce report on the diagnosis and clinical management of COVID-19 associated pulmonary aspergillosis. Intensive Care Med. 2021;47:819–34.
3. Huang L, He H, Ding Y, Jin J, Zhan Q. Values of radiological examinations for the diagnosis and prognosis of invasive bronchial-pulmonary aspergillosis in critically ill patients with chronic obstructive pulmonary diseases. Clin Respir J. 2018;12:499-509. https://doi.org/10.1111/crj.12551.
4. Lass-Flörl C. How to make a fast diagnosis in invasive aspergillosis. Med Mycol. England; 2019;57:S155–60.
5. Ullmann AJ, Aguado JM, Arikan-Akdagli S, Denning DW, Groll AH, Lagrou K, et al. Diagnosis and management of Aspergillus diseases: executive summary of the 2017 ESCMID-ECMM-ERS guideline. Clin Microbiol Infect Off Publ Eur Soc Clin Microbiol Infect Dis. England; 2018;24 Suppl 1:e1–38.
6. Garcia-Vidal C, Alastruey-Izquierdo A, Aguilar-Guisado M, Carratalà J, Castro C, Fernández-Ruiz M, et al. Executive summary of clinical practice guideline for the management of invasive diseases caused by Aspergillus: 2018 Update by the GEMICOMED-SEIMC/REIPI. Enfermedades Infecc y Microbiol Clin (English ed). Spain; 2019;37:535–41.
7. Patterson TF, Thompson GR 3rd, Denning DW, Fishman JA, Hadley S, Herbrecht R, et al. Practice Guidelines for the Diagnosis and Management of Aspergillosis: 2016 Update by the Infectious Diseases Society of America. Clin Infect Dis an Off Publ Infect Dis Soc Am. 2016;63:e1–60.

8. De Pauw B, Walsh TJ, Donnelly JP, Stevens DA, Edwards JE, Calandra T, et al. Revised definitions of invasive fungal disease from the European Organization for Research and Treatment of Cancer/Invasive Fungal Infections Cooperative Group and the National Institute of Allergy and Infectious Diseases Mycoses Study Group (EORTC/MSG) Consensus Group. Clin Infect Dis. 2008;46: 1813–21.
9. Bergeron A, Porcher R, Sulahian A, de Bazelaire C, Chagnon K, Raffoux E, et al. The strategy for the diagnosis of invasive pulmonary aspergillosis should depend on both the underlying condition and the leukocyte count of patients with hematologic malignancies. Blood. 2012;119, http://dx.doi.org/10.1182/blood-2011-04-351601, 1831-1837 [quiz 1956].
10. Acosta J, Catalan M, del Palacio-Pérez-Medel A, Montejo JC, de-La-Cruz-Bértolo J, Moragues MD, et al. Prospective study in critically ill non-neutropenic patients: Diagnostic potential of (1,3)-B-D-glucan assay and circulating galactomannan for the diagnosis of invasive fungal disease. Eur J Clin Microbiol Infect Dis. 2012;31:721–31, http://dx.doi.org/10.1007/s10096-011-1365-0.
11. Talento AF, Dunne K, Joyce EA, Palmer M, Johnson E, White PL, et al. A prospective study of fungal biomarkers to improve management of invasive fungal diseases in a mixed specialty critical care unit. J Crit Care. 2017; 40:119–27, http://dx.doi.org/10.1016/j.jcrc 2017.03.025.
12. Bulpa P, Duplaquet F, Dimopoulos G, Vogelaers D, Blot S. Invasive Pulmonary Aspergillosis in Chronic Obstructive Pulmonary Disease Exacerbations. Semin Respir Crit Care Med. United States; 2020;41:851–61.
13. Tutar N, Metan G, Koç AN, Yilmaz I, Bozkurt I, Simsek ZO, et al. Invasive pulmonary aspergillosis in patients with chronic obstructive pulmonary disease. Multidiscip Respir Med. 2013;8:59.
14. Verweij PE, Rijnders BJA, Brüggemann RJM, Azoulay E, Bassetti M, Blot S, et al. Review of influenza-associated pulmonary aspergillosis in ICU patients and proposal for a case definition: an expert opinion. Intensive Care Med. 2020;46:1524–35.
15. Chong WH, Neu KP. Incidence, diagnosis and outcomes of COVID-19-associated pulmonary aspergillosis (CAPA): a systematic review. J Hosp Infect. 2021;113:115–29.
16. Philipp Koehler, Matteo Bassetti, Arunaloke Chakrabarti, Sharon CA Chen, et al. Definición y manejo de la aspergilosis pulmonar asociada a COVID-19: los criterios de consenso ECMM/ISHAM 2020 para investigación y orientación clínica. Lancet Infect Dis. 2021 junio; 21(6): e149–e162.
17. Arastehfar A, Carvalho A, van de Veerdonk FL. COVID-19 associated pulmonary aspergillosis (CAPA)—from immunology to treatment. J Fungi (Basel) 2020; 6:91.
18. White PL, Dhillon R, Cordey A. A national strategy to diagnose COVID-19 associated invasive fungal disease in the ICU. Clin Infect Dis. 2020 doi: 10.1093/cid/ciaa1298. published online Aug 29.
19. Verweij PE, Gangneux J-P, Bassetti M. Diagnosing COVID-19-associated pulmonary aspergillosis. Lancet Microbe. 2020;1:e53–e55.
20. Bassetti M. et al, Issues in the management of invasive pulmonary aspergillosis in non-neutropenic patients in the intensive care unit: A role for isavuconazole. IDCases. 2018. 12:7–9.
21. Bassetti M. et al, Intensive care medicine research agenda on invasive fungal infection in critically ill patients. Intensive Care Med. 2017 Sep;43(9):1225–1238.
22. Walsh TJ, Anaissie EJ, Denning DW, Herbrecht R, Dimitrios P. et al. Treatment of Aspergillosis: Guidelines for Practice. Infectious Diseases Society of America (IDSA). Infectious Diseases Society of the United States (IDSA) Clinical Practice Guidelines.

CHAPTER

13

Acute Liver Failure in the ICU

Pedro Arriaga

ABSTRACT

Acute liver failure (ALF) is a rare and severe hepatic syndrome that has a diverse etiology that varies also according to geographical distribution. Clinically these patients present symptoms of jaundice, rapid development encephalopathy and coagulopathy. Important factors affecting the clinical progression of these patients in the ICU are: Early recognition, team approach and aggressive management.

■ **Keywords:** *Clinical history, team approach, medications and drug overdose, viral infections, support treatment, liver transplant.*

CASE PRESENTATION

A 44-year-old female patient presented to the Accident and Emergency Department complaining of malaise, yellow discoloration to her eyes, confusion, disorientation, mild generalized abdominal pain, nausea, vomiting and fever. The patient's husband told the doctor that his wife had just returned from Guatemala 5 days ago. On admission, physical examination revealed an acutely ill patient, pale and diaphoretic. Vital signs were: BP 80/50 mm Hg, Hr110, T 100 F, RR 25, Sat02 90% (at room air).

Patient was jaundiced, confused, disoriented but her pupils were responsive. The oral mucosa was dry, and there was no mass or adenopathy in the neck. The chest was symmetrical with use of accessory muscles, auscultation of her lungs with bilateral creps. The abdomen was soft, depressible with no hepatosplenomegaly. The patient was moving her 4 extremities. Asterixis was present. This patient had no previous medical history of any illness, allergies, no alcohol ingestion or use of illicit drugs. Labs reported a WBC of 15.0 × 109/L with the following differential: Polys 90%, lymph 10%, platelets 50,000 per microliter, creatinine 2.5 mg/dl, BUN 70 mg/dl, INR 3, fibrinogen level 90 mg/dl, bilirubin total 5.5 mg/dl, direct bilirubin 3.5 mg/dl, GOT 7000 U/L, GPT 6500 U/L, sugar level 70 mg/dl, lactate level was 4 mmol/L. Chest X-ray showed bilateral patchy infiltrates, arterial blood gases (ABGs) showed metabolic acidosis and hypoxia with a P/F ratio of 100. Blood and urinary cultures were made, serology for HIV was reported negative and serology for hepatitis A, B, C were requested. Patient blood pressure did not improved after the use of IV crystalloids. Her level of consciousness deteriorated and her respiratory distress intensified. Norepinephrine was started and she was intubated.

What diagnosis can explain the clinical presentation and progression of this patient?

This patient presented to the emergency acutely ill with alteration of the level of consciousness, respiratory problems and renal failure. She was in shock and not responding to fluids. The diagnosis of sepsis could have been a reasonable possibility considering her state of shock involving multiple organ failure. Screening for a source of infection was important (blood cultures were taken). The use of antibiotics was considered as part of the treatment.

Acute liver failure is another possibility that we needed to exclude, because of the alterations in the liver function with no previous medical history (important alterations in INR, thrombocytopenia and low levels of fibrinogen), alterations in the level of consciousness, and the presence of asterixis (although non-specific).

Because of the diverse causative variety and potential severity of ALF, a screening process should be started immediately.

DEFINITION

Acute liver failure (ALF) is an uncommon and potentially fatal syndrome from diverse etiologies with variable course and outcome that presents with jaundice, synthetic liver failure (INR >1.5, abnormal liver function tests: Elevation of transaminases >25 times the upper normal level), and hepatic encephalopathy in patients with no previous history of liver disease all within 26 weeks from the onset of illness.[1,2,3]

Classification

In 1993, O'Grady and colleagues developed the King's classification that also had the advantage of a prognostic value:

1. Hyper-acute liver failure is when encephalopathy occurs within 7 days after the onset of jaundice. This form of the disease has a better prognosis but a higher incidence of brain edema, severe coagulopathy and marked increase in transaminases.
2. Acute liver failure: Encephalopathy occurs between 8 days and 4 weeks.
3. Subacute liver failure when encephalopathy occurs within 5 weeks and 26 weeks.

Acute and sub-acute forms have worst prognosis, but lower incidence of brain edema.[3]

Another classification is the one from the International Association for the Study of the Liver (IASL):

A. Hyper-acute liver failure when encephalopathy is established in less than 10 days.
B. Fulminant when encephalopathy occurs between 10 days and 30 days.
C. Sub-acute liver failure when encephalopathy occurs between weeks 5 and 24.[4]

Epidemiology

The incidence of ALF is 1–10 cases per million inhabitants, with mortality rates of 80%. This is a condition that affects mainly young people (peak age 35–45 years and female patients (60% of cases). ALF is responsible for 6% of deaths related to liver disease and 7% to 8% of deaths of liver transplant patients.[6,7,8]

Etiology

Conditions that cause ALF have a diverse geographical variation. ALF is less common in the developed world where drug-induced liver injury is the most common cause (acetaminophen hepatic toxicity represent ~50% of cases). Acetaminophen hepatic toxicity is a dose dependent condition that can be either acute (suicidal attempts) or progressive and is rarely associated to therapeutic doses.[2,6,7]

In the developing world, the majority of cases are caused by viral infections such as: Hepatitis A, B and E with death rates of more than 50%, can be associated to low vaccination practices and poor sanitation. In critically ill patients with sepsis, acute ischemic hepatocellular injury can be a contributing factor for ALF.[9,10]

Other conditions associated with ALF are: Budd-Chiari syndrome, cytomegalovirus, Epstein-Barr virus, herpes simplex infections, HELLP syndrome, acute fatty liver of pregnancy, Wilson's disease, the use of drugs (NSAIDs, beta lactams), herbal products (mushrooms), heat stroke, cocaine use, and malignancies (breast, lungs, lymphoma). Idiosyncratic forms of ALF have been reported in up to 15% of adult patients.[2,6 7,9,10]

Clinical Signs and Symptoms

Symptoms of acute liver failure can be non-specific in early stages: Malaise, nausea, vomiting, non-specific abdominal pain. Hyper-acute cases can show confusion, disorientation, mild jaundice and a fast presentation encephalopathy.

Hepatic encephalopathy has a diverse clinical presentation and can be classified as follows:

Grade I: Mild confusion, sleeping alterations, euphoria or depression, shortened attention span

Grade II: Lethargy and moderate confusion, inappropriate behavior

Grade III: Marked confusion, gross disorientation, patient becomes drowsy

Grade IV: Coma[11]

The presence of asterixis is more common in Grade II and III but is absent in Grade IV. Electroencephalograms (EEGs) are usually normal in Grade I, but abnormal in the rest (II, III, IV).[11]

Patients with obesity, diabetes mellitus and with moderate alcohol ingestion have a higher risk for developing acute liver failure.[12,13]

Acute kidney failure can be present in 70% of cases and 30% will need renal replacement therapy. Elderly patients and patients with acetaminophen induced ALF have more risk to develop kidney failure.[12,14]

Screening

Finding the etiology of acute liver failure is critical for the management and prognosis of patients. Clinical history is very important to help and guide the diagnostic process in patients with ALF.

Clinicians should obtain the following information:

1. Use of medications and drugs (e.g. cocaine or some other form of illicit drugs),
2. Family history
3. Travel history
4. Time of jaundice in relation to symptoms
5. Blood transfusions
6. Occupation
7. Sexual contacts
8. Exposure to toxins (mushrooms, organic solvents)
9. The use of herbal or traditional medications.[13,14]

Laboratory Findings and Diagnostic Tests

Alterations in the prothrombin time with INR >1.5, elevation in liver function tests specially in the transaminases and bilirubin levels, elevated amylase and lipase levels, elevated ammonia level and hypoglycemia can be present in patients with acute liver failure. Consideration must be made for screening of blood and urine toxicology (acetaminophen, illicit drugs) and serology for viral hepatitis and HIV. Abdominal ultrasound and CT can be helpful looking for malignant infiltration, liver steatosis, occlusion of hepatic veins, portal hypertension. Liver biopsy must be considered depending of the clinical status of patients and when the initial evaluation did not identify the cause.[6,10,14,15]

Following the above case, the patient continued being hypotensive even with the use of high dose of norepinephrine, the addition of vasopressin and the addition of stress dose of steroids. Antibiotic therapy was initiated with piperacillin-tazobactan according to renal function. Mechanical ventilation was modified due to presence of ARDS with the use of low tidal volumes, FI02 and PEEP levels according to the degree of hypoxia. Serology results for hepatitis were reported positive for hepatitis B and negative for hepatitis A and C. The family was re-interviewed and they reported that this patient was born in Guatemala and migrated to the United States when she was 16 years old and was never vaccinated for hepatitis A and B. A brain CT was performed earlier and reported without abnormalities. Clinical evaluation for the presence of encephalopathy (except for the neurological changes on the arrival to the emergency) was not possible because the patient was under sedation.

Two days later despite all efforts, the patient's renal function deteriorated, she became hypoglycemic, her ABGs showed severe metabolic acidosis with refractory hypoxia, her platelets levels decreased to 10000 per microliter, she went into cardiac arrest and died.

What are the principles of management of patients with ALF?

Management

General Considerations

Patients with acute liver failure must be managed in the ICU with a systematic approach, the help of a multidisciplinary team and ideally in institutions with a liver transplant program a difficult situation especially in developing countries. These patients usually have a low intravascular volume and vasoplegia and are in need of fluid resuscitation and hemodynamic monitoring. Considerations for the use of vasopressors must be made, norepinephrine is the agent of choice and vasopressin should be the second. Cortisol deficiency has been well-reported in patients with acute liver failure and stress dose of steroids must be considered. Endotracheal intubation with mechanical ventilatory support in patients with advanced encephalopathy, shock and respiratory distress must be performed. ALF patients are hypercatabolic and hypoglycemia is very common and a sign of poor prognosis demanding early nutritional support.[14,15,16,17]

Coagulopathy

Coagulopathy can be a part of this syndrome due to the inability of the liver to synthesize clotting factors, thrombocytopenia and low levels of fibrinogen. Although INR can be elevated this will not help to assess the risk of bleeding, in some studies the use of thromboelastometry has been helpful. A state of rebalance hemostasis has been described because of a simultaneous reduction of anticoagulants (protein S, C and anti-thrombin) and elevation of von Willebrand factor. Using fresh frozen plasma has not shown changes in mortality, may increase the possibility of fluid overload and can interfere with the evaluation of the hepatic function. Preventative treatment for gastrointestinal bleeding must be initiated.[14,18,19,20]

Neurological Problems

Neurological problems can develop depending of the severity of the hepatic encephalopathy, the presence of brain edema and intracranial hypertension that correlates to high mortality (approximately 55%). In the past years there has been a reduction in the incidence of brain edema which is believed have improved due to early recognition and medical management.[14]

Risk factors for developing brain edema are: Hyperacute presentations, younger age, renal and cardiac dysfunction and elevated arterial ammonia levels (>150 umol/L).[14]

High ammonia levels can induce astrocyte swelling, mitochondrial dysfunction and glutathione related osmotic brain edema that can increase intracranial hypertension, so it is important to try to reduce the ammonia production and to increase clearance. Renal replacement therapy is an efficient way to reduce levels of ammonia. Therapy with lactulose and L-ornithine L-aspartate (LOLA) has been used in patients with acute liver with no definitive results.[14,20,21]

Seizures are common in patients with ALF and they should be closely monitored and treated once they are confirmed, the use of EEGs must be considered in patients that are ventilated, phenytoin is the drug of choice and there is no evidence that supports the use of prophylactic treatment for seizures.[22]

If intracranial hypertension is a possibility, invasive ICP monitoring or the use of transcranial Doppler, evaluation of the optic nerve sheath diameter and the use of near-infrared spectrophotometry must be considered.[14,23]

Infections

Sepsis is one of the leading causes of death in patients with ALF and is a risk factor for progression of encephalopathy. Bacterial (pneumonias and urinary tract infections) and fungal infections are common so clinicians must be performing blood and urinary cultures in these patients. There is no evidence supporting the use of prophylactic antibiotics in ALF.[17,24,25]

Specific Therapies

Acetaminophen induced hepatic toxicity:

Acetaminophen is the most common cause of ALF in the USA and Europe with 50% of cases caused by unintentional overdose and more than half of these involving opioid combination products. The mortality of patients in ALF related to acetaminophen is 28% and a third of these patients will be in need of liver transplant.[26,27]

Clinical history and measurement of acetaminophen levels will help to establish the diagnosis.

Accumulation of N-acetyl-p-benzoquinone imine (NAPQI), a product of acetaminophen metabolism through the cytochrome p-450, is associated to mitochondrial dysfunction and liver injury. Therapeutic use of N-acetylcysteine induces the production of glutathione that blocks the accumulation of this metabolite.[26,27,28]

The management of these patients relies on supportive care, prevention of drug absorption (use of activated charcoal) and the administration of antidotes (N-acetylcysteine) when applicable.[26,27,28]

ALF Related to Viral Infections

The most common cause of ALF in developing countries is viral infections, of which Hepatitis B and E are the main etiologies.

Hepatitis A tends to be a mild disease but causes severe forms of ALF. Treatment for hepatitis A and E is mainly supportive. Patients with ALF that is caused by hepatitis B infection may have the benefit of antiviral therapy, but will not prevent the need for transplant. The prognosis in patients with ALF related to hepatitis B is poor without a liver transplant and the survival rate in these patients range from 26–53%.[29,30,31]

Role of Liver Transplant

Liver transplant can be an option in some conditions that causes ALF but is not universally available. The survival rate after one year ranges from 50–79%. Approximately, 10% of all liver transplants are performed in patients with ALF.[32]

Predictive factors that help us to identify patients with worst prognosis are:

1. Etiology: Most patients with acetaminophen toxicity, hepatitis A, and ischemic hepatitis do not need a liver transplant. On the other hand, most patients with idiosyncratic forms and autoimmune diseases will need a transplant.
2. Sub-acute forms of ALF
3. The degree of encephalopathy
4. Age
5. The presence of renal failure
6. Sepsis
7. Hypoglycemia[32–33]

Prognostic models have been developed to help us identify patients with high mortality if they do not received a transplant. One of the most well-known models is the King's College Hospital Criteria. If a patient is admitted with poor prognosis, the recommendation would be to refer he or she to a transplant center if available.[32,33,34]

Contraindications for liver transplant are: Active alcohol abuse, advance age brain death active infection and uncontrolled sepsis, severe cardiopulmonary disease, extra-hepatic malignancy with metastases.[35,36]

REFERENCES

1. Bower WA et al Population based surveillance for acute liver failure Am Grastroenterol 2007; 102:2459–63.
2. Lai W K et al Management of acute failure. Continuing Education in Anesthesia Critical Care and Pain 2004 Vol 4, No 2 40–43.
3. O'Grady JG et al. Acute Liver Failure: redefining the syndrome. Lancet 1993:342: 273–5.
4. Tandon BN et al Recommendations of the international Association for the study of the liver subcommittee on nomenclature of acute and subacute liver failure. J Gastroenterol Hepato 1999: 14: 403–404.
5. European Association for the Study of the Liver. EASL Clinical practical guidelines on the management of acute (fulminant) liver failure. Journal of Hepatology 2017 Vol 66: 1047–1081.
6. Bernal W et al. Acute liver failure NEJM 2012 396:26 2525–34.
7. Ostapowicz et al. Results of a prospective study of acute liver failure at 17 tertiary care centers in the United States Ann Intern Med 2002 Dec 17; 137(12): 947–54.
8. Lee WM et al. Acute Liver Failure: Summary of workshop. Hepatology2008 Apr: 47(4): 1401–1415.
9. Reuben A et al. Drug induced acute liver failure results of U.S. multicenter prospective study. Hepatology 2010; 52: 2065–76.

10. Seetheram A. Intensive care management of acute liver failure considerations while awaiting liver transplantation J Clin Transl Hepatology 2019 Dec 28 7(4)384–91.
11. Ferenci P et al. Hepatic encephalopathy—definition, nomenclature, diagnosis and quantification: final report of the working party at the 11th World Congresses of gastroenterology, Vienna, 1998. Hepatology, 2002; 35; 716–21.
12. Bernal W et al. Acute Liver Failure. N Engl J Med 2013: 369: 2525–34.
13. Vasquez F et al. Acute liver failure. Critical Care vol 28 (2) April 2022: 198–207.
14. Trujios SR et al. Risk factors and outcomes of acute kidney injury in patients with acute liver failure. Clin Gastroenterol hepatol. 2015; 13(2): 352–9.
15. Gill RQ et al. Acute liver failure. J Clin Gastroenterol. 2001 33 (3); 191–8.
16. Aziz R et al. Management of acute liver failure in intensive care. BJA education January 2021;21 (3): 110–16.
17. Priyanka R R et al. Management of acute liver failure in the intensive care unit setting. Clinics in liver disease vol 22 (2) May 2018: 403–408.
18. Agarwal B et al. Evaluation of coagulation abnormalities in acute liver failure. J HEPATOL 2012; 57: 780–6.
19. Lissman T et al. the concept of rebalanced hemostasis in patients with liver disease: Communication from the ISTH SSC working group on hemostatic management of patients with liver disease. J Thromb Hemost 2021; 19: 1116–1122.
20. Munoz SJ et al. Coagulopathy of acute liver failure. Clin Liver Dis 2009; 13 (1): 95.
21. Acharya et al. Efficacy of L-Ornithine L-aspartate in acute liver failure: a double blind, randomized, placebo control study Gastroenterology 2009; 136: 2159–2168.
22. Ellis AJ et al. Subclinical seizure activity and prophylactic phenytoin infusion in acute liver failure: a control clinical trial. Hepatology 2000; 32(3); 536.
23. Sheikh MF et al. Neurological monitoring in acute liver failure J Clin Exp Hepatol 2018; 8: 441–7.
24. Rolando N et al. Bacterial and fungal infection in acute liver failure. Semin Liver Dis 1996; 16: 389–402.
25. Rolando et al. The systemic inflammatory response syndrome in acute liver failure. Hepatology. 2000; 32 734–9.
26. Lieden M et al. A perspective on the epidemiology of acetaminophen exposure and toxicity in the United States. Expert Rev Clin Pharmacol 2014; 7(3): 341.
27. Lancaster E et al. Acetaminophen hepatotoxicity: and updated review ArchToxicol 2015; 89:193–9.
28. Lee WM. Drug induced hepatotoxicity. N Engl J Med 2003;349 (5): 474.
29. Manka P et al. Liver Failure due to Acute Viral hepatitis (A-E)Visc Med 2016 Apr; 32 (2): 80–5.
30. Belongia EA et al. NIH consensus development statement on management of hepatitis B. NIH Consent State Sci statements 2008: 25 (2):1.
31. Lee HC et al. Acute liver failure related to hepatitis B virus. Hepatol Res. 2008; 38 (suppl 1) S9–S13.
32. NHS Blood and transplant. Annual report on liver transplantation: report for 2019.
33. Castaldo ET et al. Liver transplantation for acute hepatic failure. HPB Journal 2006; 8: 29–34.
34. Hoofnagle JH et al. Fulminant hepatic failure: summary of a workshop. Hepatology 1995; 21:240–52.
35. O'Grady JG et al. Early indicators of prognosis in fulminant hepatic failure. Gastroenterology. 198; 97: 439–45.
36. Varma V et al. Indications and contraindications for liver transplant. International Journal of Hepatology artcle 2011 ID 121862 1–9.

CHAPTER

14

Delirium

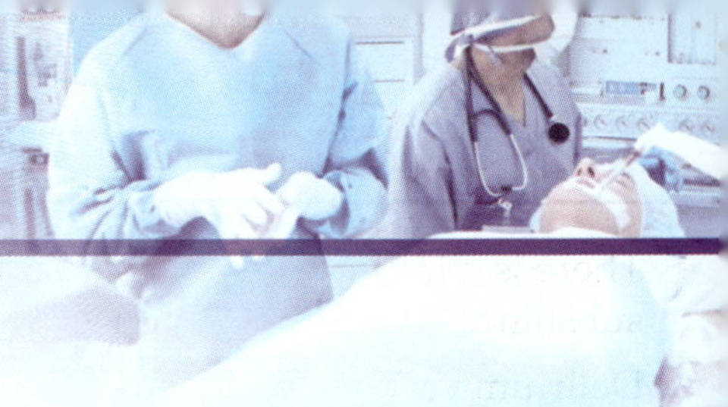

Monika Gulati

CLINICAL VIGNETTE

A 40-year-old diabetic man has been admitted in ICU for 4 days after undergoing emergency laparotomy for a perforated duodenal ulcer. He had a delayed admission to the hospital due to staying at a far distance from the hospital. Intraoperatively he was found to have 4 quadrant soiling of the abdomen with feculent peritonitis. He was sedated and mechanically ventilated in ICU with fentanyl and midazolam infusion with ongoing vasopressor support for hemodynamic instability. During the last 4 days he received CRRT for oliguric AKI. Weaning trials were attempted post-stabilization and he has been extubated today. He was very agitated on the ventilator. After 8 hours of extubation he is drowsy but responsive to verbal commands with a GCS of 14. His vitals are: HR: 110/min, afebrile, BP: 110/70 mm Hg without vasopressor support, RR: 18/min, O_2 sats: 95–97% on nasal cannula@ 3 L/min.

Standard Approach to Management

What are the possible causes of this patient's fluctuating consciousness?

The fluctuation in consciousness of this patient is characterized by agitation and drowsiness in a short span of time which is very typical of mixed delirium. Various factors that can contribute to this include pain, hypo/hyperglycemia, electrolyte imbalances, ongoing sepsis, uraemia and a possibility of any neurological event like stroke.These need to be ruled out by a thorough systemic examination and reviewing the blood tests. Hypoxia and underperfusion of the brain are possible but in this case both hemodynamics and respiratory parameters of the patient do not indicate that.

What is delirium and how common is this condition in critically ill patients?

Delirium is a serious but often overlooked and unrecognized condition that might occur in critically ill patients. According to the DSM-5 (Diagnostic and Statistical Manual of Mental Disorders Fifth Edition), delirium includes the presence of all of the following criteria:

- Disturbance in attention such as to direct, focus, sustain and shift attention and awareness, i.e. orientation to the environment occuring acutely and the severity tends to fluctuate over the course of the day.
- Disturbed cognition—any one of memory deficit, disorientation, language, visuospatial ability, perception.
- The above are not explained by pre-existing illness such as dementia or not occurring during the course of arousal from coma.

- There is clinical evidence of an underlying organic cause such as a medical condition or substance abuse.[1,2]

Delirium varies in incidence from 15% to 85%. Elderly population in medical and surgical ICUs, 15 to 25% patients after major elective surgery and 50% patients after high-risk orthopedic and cardiac surgeries experience delirium. The prevalence among palliative care patients reaches as high as 85%.[3,4] The diagnosis of delirium is clinical, with no specific laboratory or imaging tests available to detect it. A clinical index of suspicion along with regular monitoring of ICU patients with clinical monitoring tools for early identification and treatment of delirium are recommended.

What are the types of delirium?

There are various ways of classifying delirium but the most common way is dependent on how it manifests clinically: Hyperactive (agitation, restlessness), hypoactive (apathy, drowsiness) and mixed (fluctuation between the two forms). Hypoactive delirium is not only difficult to diagnose but is also associated with worse prognosis.[5] If one or more of the delirium criteria are not met, it is called subsyndromal delirium.[6] The clinical phenotypes of delirium have also been classified depending on etiology as hypoxic, septic, sedative-associated, or metabolic (renal or liver dysfunction) delirium.

What is the relation between the different clinical phenotypes of delirium and outcome?

Two studies MIND-ICU[7] and BRAIN-ICU[8] evaluated the relation of type of clinical phenotype to cognitive function at 12 months using the RBANS score. These studies showed that delirium associated with prolonged sedation, hypoxia and sepsis had the worst cognitive outcomes at the end of 12 months.

What are the potential causes/contributing factors leading to development of delirium?

Delirium is a multifactorial disorder. A number of factors may collectively contribute to the condition, some may increase the baseline susceptibility or may precipitate the state.

Non-modifiable factors:

Older age

Prior cognitive impairment: Dementia/psychiatric disorders, Parkinson's disease

Hypertension

Neurologic disease

High severity of illness on admission: High APACHE and ASA scores

Pre-ICU emergency surgery or trauma

Antipsychotic/anticonvulsant use

Postoperative states specially in elderly patients

Modifiable factors

Benzodiazepine infusions, e.g. Midazolam, Lorazepam. (Strong evidence)[9]

Blood transfusions (Strong evidence)[9]

Pain

Isolation

Indwelling catheters

Ongoing sepsis

Multiorgan failure

Fluid and electrolyte imbalances (hypo/hypernatremia, dehydration)
Long stay in ICU/on ventilator
Immobility
Physical restraints
Sleep deprivation
Disorientation, e.g. lack of hearing aids/eyeglasses
Nicotine use
Drug or alcohol abuse/withdrawal from alcohol, Benzodiazepines, Barbiturates or SSRIs.

How can delirium be detected in a timely fashion to prevent worse outcomes?

Confusion Assessment Method for the ICU (CAM-ICU) or the Intensive Care Delirium Screening Checklist (ICDSC) are the scoring systems that can be utilized for early recognition of delirium by trained and experienced ICU nurses as recommended by the 2018 Pain, Agitation/Sedation, Delirium, Immobility, and Sleep Disruption in Adult Patients in the ICU (PADIS) Guidelines.[9]

Both these instruments score high in the inter-rater reliability, however, the specificity of CAM-ICU is 89–93%, whereas that of ICDSC is only 64%. They can be used for both the diagnosis of delirium and monitoring the evolution of delirium that may otherwise go unnoticed. The CAM-ICU score is one of the most widely used scores for assessment of delirium in ICU.[10]

Flowchart 14.1: Confusion assessment method-the intensive care unit (CAM-ICU)[10]

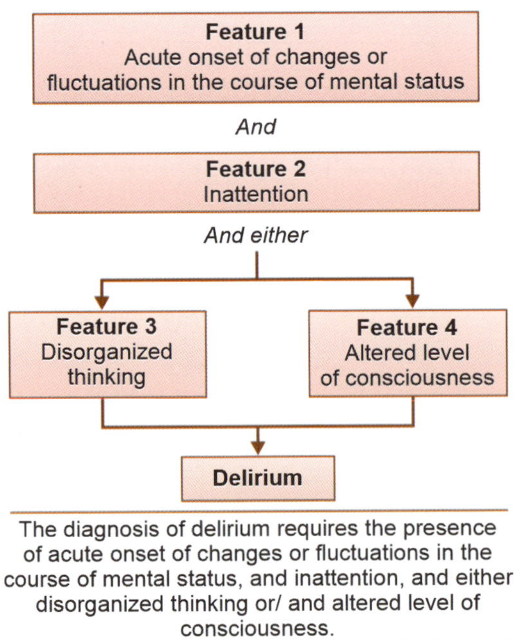

A new severity assessment tool (the CAM-ICU-7) available for documenting severity of delirium is available and this is important because increasing severity is associated with poorer outcome.[11] This score ranges from 0 to 7 and is subcategorized into 0–2: No delirium, 3–5: Mild to moderate delirium, and 6–7: Severe delirium.

Table 14.1: CAM-ICU-7 Delirium severity scale[11]

CAM-ICU		
Items	***Grading***	***Score***
1. Acute onset or fluctuation of mental status Is the patient different than his/her baseline mental status? OR Has the patient had any fluctuation in mental status in the past 24 hours as evidenced by fluctuation on a sedation/level of consciousness scale (i.e. RASS/SAS), GCS, or previous delirium assessment?	0 absent 1 present	
2. Inattention Say to the patient, "I am going to read you a series of 10 letters. Whenever you hear the letter 'A', indicate by squeezing my hand". Read letters from the following letter list in a normal tone 3 seconds apart. <u>SAVEAHAART</u> (Errors are counted when patient fails to squeeze on the letter "A" and when the patient squeezes on any letter other than "A")	0 absent (correct ≥8) 1 for inattention (correct 4–7) 2 for severe inattention (correct 0–3)	
3. Altered level of consciousness Present if the actual RASS score is anything other than alert and calm (zero)	0 absent (RASS 0) 1 for altered level (RASS 1, –1) 2 for severe altered level (RASS >1, <–1)	
4. Disorganized thinking Yes/No questions 1. Will a stone float on water? 2. Are there fish in the sea? 3. Does one pound weight more than two pounds? 4. Can you use a hammer to pound a nail? Errors are counted when the patient incorrectly answers a question. Command: Say to patient "Hold up this many fingers" (Hold two fingers in front of patient). "Now do the same with the other hand" (Do not repeat number of fingers) An error is counted if patient is unable to complete the entire command.	0 absent (correct ≥4) 1 for disorganized thinking (correct 2, 3) 2 for severe diorganized thinking (correct 0, 1)	
	Total score	

CAM-ICU: Confusion Assessment Method for the Intensive Care Unit; RASS: Richmond Agitation Sedation Scale; SAS: Sedation-Agitation Scale; GCS: Glasgow Coma Scale.

What is the Differential Diagnosis of Delirium?

It is important to differentiate delirium from other psychotic or neurological disorders. However, the distinct clinical features of delirium with acute and fluctuating course help in making diagnosis easier. Since a lot of medical disorders can cause delirium, it is imperative to rule out these organic causes.

Some important differentials to be considered are:

- Dementia (chronic, insidious, progressive and without much fluctuations)
- NCSE
- Primary psychiatric illnesses (depression, mania, schizophrenia).

How can delirium be prevented in a patient admitted in ICU?

Prevention of delirium in ICU should be a multi-model approach with focus on modifiable risk factors.

This approach includes:

1. Nonpharmacological interventions[9, 12–16]
2. Sedation protocols/avoidance of drugs causing delirium.

1. Nonpharmacological interventions: A multidisciplinary approach is helpful that includes:
   - Early mobilization of patients (active physiotherapy, exercise and mental stimulation of patients during the daytime).
   - Minimized use of physical restraints in patients.
   - Day/night orientation: Ensuring adequate and good quality sleep by avoiding excessive noise by nursing staff at nighttime, and keeping lights dim at night.
   - Provision of aids: Visual/hearing to assist the special needs.
   - Allowing family members at regular intervals in daytime for cognitive stimulation.
   - Reorientation by medical staff and family by introduction, talking about the events and using a clock may all be helpful techniques.
2. Sedation protocols in ICU and avoidance of drugs causing delirium: These interventions include physician and nurse driven appropriate sedation protocols in ICU for both mechanically ventilated and non-ventilated patients.
   - Appropriate sedation using sedation scores (with a goal of calm and arousable patient: RASS score 0/–1, and avoidance of a either a too combative/drowsy patient)
   - Daily sedation vacation
   - Avoidance of benzodiazepine infusions for sedation: Benzodiazepine infusions should be avoided unless the patient has concerns of alcohol withdrawal
   - Use of dexmedetomidine/propofol for sedation in ventilated patients
   - Adequate pain management
   - Addressing background etiologies of ICU admission like infection, hypoxemia.

What drug can be used to prevent delirium in critically ill surgical and medical patients?

There are no drugs recommended to prevent delirium in the ICU.[9]

What are the harmful effects of delirium if left untreated?

Short-term complications

- Potential self-extubation and loss of airway, removal of NIV/oxygen: Leading to hypoxia
- Removal of lines and catheters leading to loss of monitoring access and risk of cardiovascular compromise
- Risks of falls, injuries
- Increased nursing manpower utilization to ensure safety of the patient
- Uncomfortable for family members to see leading to distress and dissatisfaction for the care provided by the ICU team
- Patients with hypoactive delirium may become overly drowsy leading to more investigations/neuroimaging and diagnostic tests adding to overall cost burdens
- Sympathetic stimulation causing hypertension and tachycardia contributing to the risk of myocardial ischemia in high risk elderly patients.

Long-term Complications[17–20]

- Increases the development of long-term cognitive dysfunction at 3 and 6 months post-discharge[8,18,19]
- Association with longer stay in the hospital[17, 20]
- Increased cost of care to the patient/health system.

Studies have shown that delirium is NOT consistently associated with ICU LOS, discharge destination, functional outcomes or mortality.

What are the drug therapies available for treatment of hyperactive delirium?

Typical antipsychotics: Haloperidol
Atypical antipsychotics: Quetiapine, ziprasidone, Olanzipine
Alpha-2 agonists: Dexmedetomidine is an excellent drug for management of delirium as it can be given in an infusion form, and is therefore titratable to patients' consciousness. Boluses should be avoided to prevent bradycardia.

Evidence-Controversies in Management of Delirium

1. *Use of Physical Restraints*

Physical restraints are commonly used in ICUs for critically ill adults with a pretext that it is for patient safety and helps to prevent events such as self-extubation, device removal, self-harm, injuries and falls, as well as protect staff from combative patients. However, in modern critical care practice, with the availability of effective medications to keep a patient calm and tranquil, the use of physical restraints in ICU is controversial. No RCTs have addressed this issue.

A few observational descriptive studies have reported higher incidence of events with use of physical restraints.[21,22]

The benefits/risks of restraints and drugs have to be weighed carefully and prescribed on an individual basis.

2. *Pharmacological Agents*

Haloperidol and antipsychotics

There is no drug which has evidence that it treats the underlying delirium, therefore, our attention must be paid to the individual risk factors, along with preventive strategies. Routine use of haloperidol, atypical antipsychotics like Olanzapine, quetiapine or a HMG-CoA reductase inhibitor, i.e a statin is not recommended to treat delirium.[9]

Having said that, in a hyperactive delirious state with significant anxiety, hallucinations, risk of self harm or deleterious effects, short-term use of antipsychotic medications may be beneficial.

The exact choice of drug depends on local availability, affordability and consideration to the side effects of the drugs and patient profile. It is also imperative that patients who are started on an antipsychotic drug or alpha-2 agonist for hyperactive delirium must have discontinued before discharge from the hospital to avoid morbidity and unnecessary financial cost.[9]

Dexmedetomidine

A systematic review[23] found that dexmedetomidine did reduce the incidence and duration of delirium, however, whether it actually treated it was unclear. Dexmedetomidine was compared to haloperidol in a small RCT and was found to be associated with shorter time to extubation, but this needs to be confirmed in a larger blinded RCT. However, multiple studies have shown that dexmedetomidine when compared to midazolam/lorazepam reduced the incidence and duration of delirium. Dexmedetomidine is the preferred choice when there is difficulty in weaning and liberation among agitated is recommended for delirium in mechanically ventilated patients especially when agitation is precluding weaning/extubation.[9]

3. *Nonpharmacological Interventions*

The revised awakening and breathing coordination, delirium monitoring/management, and early exercise/mobility along with family engagement (ABCDEF) bundle, was evaluated in a larger, multicenter, before-after, cohort study, and where delirium was also assessed using the CAM-ICU, an adjusted analysis showed that improvements in bundle compliance were significantly associated with reduced mortality and more ICU days without coma or delirium.[24]

Can promoting good quality sleep prevent or treat delirium?

Sleep disruption has been hypothesized to contribute to ICU delirium. The amount of REM sleep was significantly lower in patients with delirium. Days with delirium were greater in those patients having a very low amount of REM sleep suggesting a possible association between the two. Ear plug use reduced delirium and improved subjective sleep quality in a RCT.[25]

The recent PADIS guidelines recommend multicomponent strategy to promote good quality sleep based on low quality evidence, which includes noise and light reduction strategy. Propofol infusions are not recommended to promote good quality sleep. There is insufficient evidence to recommend/refute dexmedetomidine or melatonin to improve sleep.[9]

To summarize management of delirium requires teamwork involving multiple disciplines. Using multicomponent interventions seem common sense and is an evidence-based strategy, also reflecting the multifactorial nature of delirium. Future research is needed to understand the qualitative experience of delirium of the patient and the role of nonpharmacological interventions in reducing the incidence of delirium.

REFERENCES

1. American Psychiatric Association (2013) Diagnostic and statistical manual of mental disorders: DSM-5. American Psychiatric Association.
2. Slooter AJC, Otte WM, Devlin JW, Arora RC, Bleck TP, Claassen J, Duprey MS, Ely EW, Kaplan PW, Latronico N et al (2020) Updated nomenclature of delirium and acute and encephalopathy: statement of ten Societies. Intensive Care Med 46(5):1020–1022.
3. Edward R. Marcantonio. Delirium in Hospitalized Older Adults. M.D. N Engl J Med. 2017 October 12; 377(15):1456–1466.
4. Slooter AJ, Van De Leur RR, Zaal IJ: Delirium in critically ill patients. Handb Clin Neurol 2017; 141:449–466.
5. Joanna L. Stollings, Katarzyna Kotfs, Gerald Chanques, Brenda T. Pun, Pratik P. Pandharipande and E. Wesley Ely Delirium in critical illness: clinical manifestations, outcomes, and management. Intensive Care Med (2021) 47:1089–1103.
6. Ouimet S, Riker R, Bergeron N, et al: Subsyndromal delirium in the ICU: Evidence for a disease spectrum. Intensive Care Med 2007;33:1007–1013.
7. Girard T D, Exline M C, Carson S S, Hough C L,Rock P et al. Haloperidol and Ziprasidone for Treatment of Delirium in Critical Illness, for the MIND-USA investigators. N Engl J Med. 2018 December 27; 379 (26) : 2506–2516.

8. Pandharipande PP, Girard TD, Jackson JC, Morandi A, Thompson JL, Pun BT, Brummel NE, Hughes CG, Vasilevskis EE, Shintani AK et al (2013) Long-term cognitive impairment after critical illness.
9. John W D,Yoanna S,Gélinas C, Dale M et al. Clinical Practice Guidelines for the Prevention and Management of Pain, Agitation/Sedation, Delirium, Immobility, and Sleep Disruption in Adult Patients in the ICU; Critical Care Medicine: September 2018 Volume 46 issue Number 9.
10. Wesley et al. Delirium in mechanically ventilated patients. Validity and reliability of the Confusion assessment method for the Intensive care Unit (CAM-ICU). JAMA,December 5, 2001,Volume 286, no. 21.
11. Babar A. Khan, MD, MS1,2,3, Anthony J. Perkins. The CAM-ICU-7 Delirium Severity Scale: A Novel Delirium Severity Instrument for Use in the Intensive Care Unit. Crit Care Med. 2017 May ; 45(5): 851–857.
12. Hoyer EH, Friedman M, Lavezza A, et al: Promoting mobility and reducing length of stay in hospitalized general medicine patients: A quality-improvement project. J Hosp Med 2016; 11:341–347391.
13. Brummel NE, Girard TD, Ely EW, et al: Feasibility and safety of early combined cognitive and physical therapy for critically ill medical and surgical patients: The Activity and Cognitive Therapy in ICU (ACT-ICU) trial. Intensive Care Med 2014; 40:370–379.
14. Colombo R, Corona A, Praga F, et al: A reorientation strategy for reducing delirium in the critically ill. Results of an interventional study. Minerva Anestesiol 2012; 78:1026–1033.
15. Hanison J, Conway D: A multifaceted approach to prevention of delirium in intensive care. BMJ Qual Improv Rep 2015; 12:4–12.
16. Rivosecchi RM, Kane-Gill SL, Svec S, et al: The implementation of a nonpharmacologic protocol to prevent intensive care delirium. J Crit Care 2016; 31:206–211.
17. Mehta S, Cook D, Devlin JW, et al; SLEAP Investigators; Canadian Critical Care Trials Group: Prevalence, risk factors, and outcomes of delirium in mechanically ventilated adults. Crit Care Med 2015; 43:557–566.
18. Wolters AE, van Dijk D, Pasma W, et al: Long-term outcome of delirium during intensive care unit stay in survivors of critical illness: A prospective cohort study. Crit Care 2014; 18:R125.
19. Girard TD, Jackson JC, Pandharipande PP, et al: Delirium as a predictor of long-term cognitive impairment in survivors of critical illness. Crit Care Med 2010; 38:1513–1520.
20. Ely EW, Gautam S, Margolin R, et al: The impact of delirium in the intensive care unit on hospital length of stay. Intensive Care Med 2001; 27:1892–1900.
21. Chang LY, Wang KW, Chao YF: Influence of physical restraint on unplanned extubation of adult intensive care patients: A case-control study. Am J Crit Care 2008; 17:408–415; quiz 416.
22. Rose L, Burry L, Mallick R, et al: Prevalence, risk factors, and outcomes associated with physical restraint use in mechanically ventilated adults. J Crit Care 2016; 31:31–35,
23. Lewis, K., Alshamsi, F., Carayannopoulos, K.L. et al. Dexmedetomidine vs other sedatives in critically ill mechanically ventilated adults: a systematic review and meta-analysis of randomized trials. Intensive Care Med 48, 811–840 (2022). https://doi.org/10.1007/s00134-022-06712-2
24. Barnes-Daly MA, Phillips G, Ely EW: Improving hospital survival and reducing brain dysfunction at seven California community hospitals: Implementing PAD guidelines via the ABCDEF bundle in 6,064 patients. Crit Care Med 2017; 45:171–178.
25. Van Rompaey B, Elseviers MM, Van Drom W, et al: The effect of earplugs during the night on the onset of delirium and sleep perception: A randomized controlled trial in intensive care patients. Crit Care 2012; 16:R73.

CHAPTER

15

Bleeding Disorders in the ICU

Angel Augusto Pérez Calatayud

CASE

A 33-year-old pregnant woman with a history of pre-eclampsia enters a c-section; the surgical team reports a 4000 ml of blood loss. A decision to perform a total hysterectomy is made, and she is admitted to the ICU. Vasopressor therapy infusion of norepinephrine 0.6 μg/kg/min and vasopressin 0.6 Ui/hr with a MAP of 37 mmHg FC 110, with an anion gap metabolic acidosis, with a lactate of 5.7 intraoperative treatment a transfusion of 3 RBC and two units of FFP were given. Administration of 4500 ml of crystalloids and colloids 150 ml albumin. Viscoelastic testing reported.

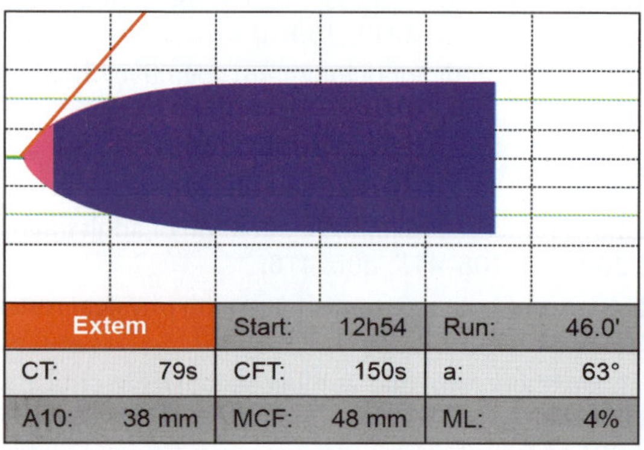

Extem		Start:	12h54	Run:	46.0'
CT:	79s	CFT:	150s	a:	63°
A10:	38 mm	MCF:	48 mm	ML:	4%

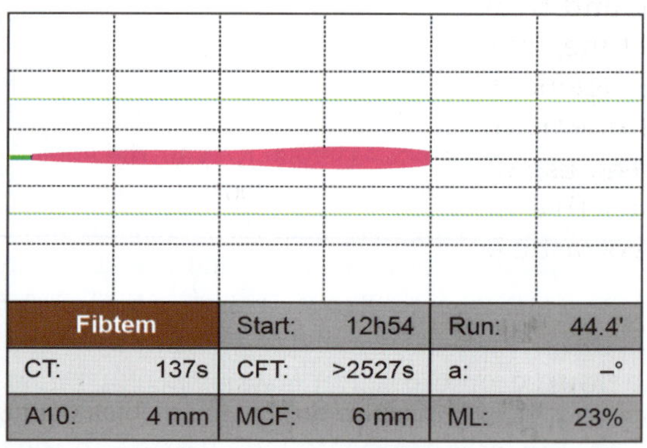

Fibtem		Start:	12h54	Run:	44.4'
CT:	137s	CFT:	>2527s	a:	–°
A10:	4 mm	MCF:	6 mm	ML:	23%

What is the Proper Management of Blood Loss and Bleeding Disorders?

Ans: In this case, a few insights of management were missed opportunities for proper treatment, which would help avoid unnecessary transfusion.

1. Bleeding source control could not be achieved, and a prolonged surgery with massive blood loss was observed.
2. At no moment was tranexamic acid used
3. Viscoelastic test results were available. There were no fibrinogen substitutions despite the evidence of active bleeding and hypofibrinogenemia.

This patient received point of care diagnostic and directed goal therapy of coagulation as soon as she arrived at the ICU. Ultrasound-guided hemodynamic management showed depleted intravascular volume, so a combination of crystalloids and colloids was used once the fluid response was assessed. After this management, the bleeding stopped, vasopressors were suspended within the day, and weaning from MV achieve within one day.

POC viscoelastic testing helped to guide coagulation management. The second test showed hyperfibrinolysis and hypofibrinogenemia. This patient was administered 1000 mg of tranexamic acid and 6 gm of fibrinogen concentrate. One more RBC was transfused, and a control thromboelastometry showed normalized parameters.

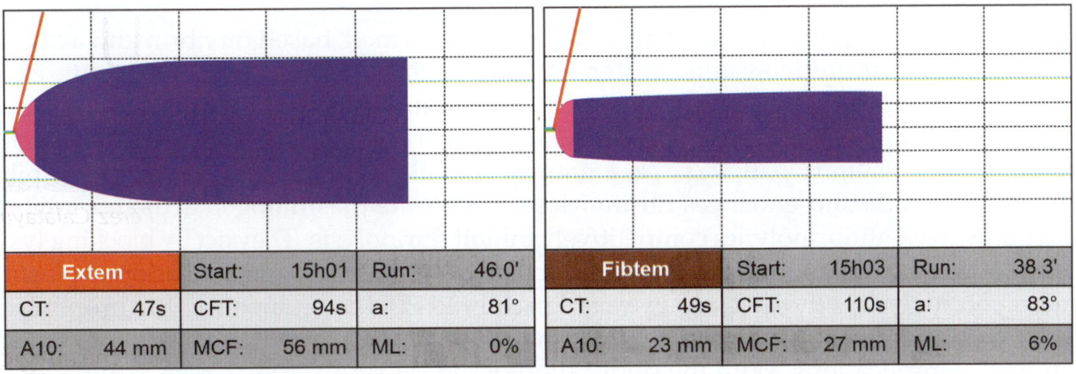

After treatment, the patients had a 3-day ICU length of stay without any further complications and did not receive any other transfusion.

PRINCIPLES OF MANAGEMENT

Bleeding patients is always challenging because there is a universal need to understand each risk and treatment approach, depending on the underlying pathology. However, most of the time, treatment management in this scenario, the transposed knowledge of transfusion management in trauma without this being evidence-based for other scenarios (such as PPH, perioperative bleeding, cardiac surgery, and liver transplant, among others).[1]

The use of algorithms of bleeding management recommended have been focusing on restrictive transfusion strategies, coagulation management, and, when available, POC viscoelastic testing.[1]

1. Bleeding Control

The source of bleeding control must be managed in the first hour (preferably in the first 30 minutes when possible),[2] this will help to avoid blood loss and coagulopathy. The location of the bleeding is essential. Bleeding control of the abdomen can be accomplished by packing and using hemostatic agents, but it requires surgical capabilities.[3] Definitive treatment of abdominopelvic bleeding often requires surgical intervention.[3] A resuscitative thoracotomy (RT) with aortic cross-clamping can be performed if a patient continues to exsanguinate despite other efforts. If available, angiographic embolization using a resuscitative endovascular balloon occlusion of the aorta (REBOA) could help to stop uncontrolled bleeding not manageable with other means. Published studies have found no difference in overall mortality between RT and REBOA.[4] The ischemia caused by occluding the aorta is one of the most significant complications for both procedures. Local hemostatic agents also help to avoid any further blood loss.[2–4]

2. Damage Control Reanimation

Damage control resuscitation has been popularized over the years because of the evidence of trauma-related coagulopathy. Treatment includes a transfusion ratio of 1:1:1 or 1:1:2 using platelets, FFP, and RBC during the reanimation. Published evidence has reported increased survival in trauma patients. However, this could lead to over-transfusion in other scenarios and should be avoided.[3]

Antifibrinolytics

Tranexamic and ε-aminocaproic acid. Once the clot is formed, based on fibrin and activated platelets, the fibrinolytic system is started in opposition to the previous one to avoid thrombosis. The presence of tissue hypoperfusion, secondary to blood loss, can lead to an upregulation of thrombomodulin, a thrombin receptor. This receptor interacts with thrombin, activating the protein C pathway. As a natural coagulant, protein C irreversibly inhibits factors Va and VIIa and enhances fibrinolysis through the plasminogen activator inhibitor (PAI) pathway. Antifibrinolytics competitively inhibit fibrinolysis. They act by blocking lysine binding sites on plasminogen molecules, which prevent plasminogen activation to plasmin. Limiting fibrinolysis is the first step in treating acquired PPH coagulopathy. The prophylactic use of tranexamic acid (TA) at doses of 1 gram or 10 to 15 mg/kg reduces blood loss without significant complications. With the publication of the WOMAN trial, Crash 2, and Crash 3 studies, Tranexamic acid is now the first-line treatment in case of substantial bleeding; one gram of TXA should be given, and an extra dose is used in case of continuous bleeding.[1–3]

Fibrinogen Concentrate for Bleeding Management

Fibrinogen (coagulation factor I) is present in the blood with an expected value of 2.0 to 4.5 g/dL. During the activation of coagulation, thrombin converts fibrinogen to fibrin polymers, forming the supporting base of the clot. A low fibrinogen level or a reduction in its function causes severe dysfunction of hemostasis. Fibrinogen can be substituted with FFP, cryoprecipitates, or fibrinogen concentrate.[3–5]

In contrast to FFP and cryoprecipitates, viral inactivation of fibrinogen concentrate is included in the manufacturing process, so the risk of transmission is minimal. Also, the fibrinogen concentration is standardized, and volume administration is low and can be used without delay because it does not require thawing. Fibrinogen concentrate has proven effective and well-tolerated in different clinical settings. The risk of thrombosis in 22 years of pharmacovigilance is low, and it has a higher efficacy profile compared to PFC.[5]

Prothrombin Complex Concentrate

Prothrombin complex concentrate (PCC) is a purified drug with hemostatic activity derived from a pooled plasma. It began to be used for clinical purposes in the 1970s as a source of factor IX to treat patients with hemophilia B.[6] The first commercially obtained PCCs contained three or four factors (factors II, IX, and X for three-factor PCC and factor VII for four-factor PCC in small portions). PCCs are mainly indicated to reverse the effects of vitamin K antagonists (acenocoumarin and warfarin). An indication that has shown a superior effect to fresh frozen plasma (FFP) by reducing the transfusion/bleeding rate in patients with active bleeding who were under treatment with these components and who required procedures.[6,7] PCC induces a rapid and effective formation of large amounts of thrombin and, subsequently, fibrinogen at the site of damage and hemostasis due to deficiency of vitamin K-dependent coagulation factors, favoring INR normalization (<1.3) over time. Of prothrombin if it is administered at an adequate dose. This reversal effect caused by CCP is faster and more complete than when PFC is administered. In different trials, it has been observed that the effect of reversing hemostasis by the FFP assessed by the INR is dose-dependent but not linear since the standard

FFP doses (15–20 ml/kg) achieve a significant reduction in the INR. However, the infusion of a larger volume of FFP (30 ml/kg) is unnecessary. The differences between CPPs and FFP could be summarized by noting that CPPs provide more complete reversal effects. They are immediately available (no crossmatching or thawing required) and are entirely safe, as they do not induce transfusion-induced lung injury and can be administered faster.[6,8]

Desmopressin

Desmopressin (DDAVP) is a rapid-acting vasopressin analog that induces in the endothelium the release of large von Willebrand factor multimers from Weibel-Palade bodies,[9] and it can be administrated intranasal, intravenous (IV) or subcutaneous (SC).

In patients with mild hemophilia A and milder forms of von Willebrand disease (VWD), DDAVP has minimized bleeding in the perioperative setting. DDAVP also promotes hemostasis in patients with uremic platelet dysfunction, although no extensive, randomized studies have demonstrated this benefit.

From a mechanistic perspective, it has been used as a non-specific hemostatic agent in patients with thrombocytopenia, as DDVAP increases circulating von Willebrand factor (VWF) and could theoretically improve platelet adhesion.

A small, randomized trial of cirrhotic patients with thrombocytopenia undergoing dental extraction demonstrated no difference between desmopressin and platelet transfusion in reducing bleeding events, but only one bleeding event occurred in the trial population, rendering a comparison of efficacy impossible.[9]

Despite the lack of evidence, DDVAP is used as a non-specific hemostatic agent in surgical patients who are uremic or refractory to platelet transfusions, and it has been reported to be well-tolerated.

Since tachyphylaxis develops quickly, DDVAP is recommended for short periods secondary to the depletion of VWF, and serum sodium should be monitored as hyponatremia is the most common complication.[9]

Point of Care Viscoelastic Testing

When available goal-directed coagulation management is associated with the viscoelastic test, the aims of ROTEM-guided bleeding management algorithms are administering the proper hemostatic intervention(s), in the correct dose, at the right time ("Treat first what kills first!"), and in the correct sequence.[9] The first step is the presence of clinically relevant bleeding and blood loss and the potential need for blood transfusion. The second and third steps deal with specific issues, such as fibrinolysis management with antifibrinolytics and anticoagulation reversal in cardiovascular surgery or heparin-like situations.

The following steps involve clot firmness management (fibrinogen and platelet transfusion). If FIBTEM clot firmness amplitude (A5 or A10, respectively) is ok, EXTEM CT can be interpreted adequately since a fibrinogen deficiency is most often associated with a prolonged EXTEM CT.[9,10,12]

ROTEM results require proper sequence in interpreting A5 before CT (amplitude after 5 minutes before coagulation time).[11,12] This avoids misinterpretation and FFP or PCC overuse, as CT may correct after fibrinogen supplementation. The other reason that clots firmness management (FIBTEM A5 and EXTEM A5) comes before thrombin generation management (EXTEM CT and INTEM CT) is that fibrinogen concentration drop-down first in severe bleeding before thrombin generation is affected (except in bleeding due to anticoagulants or hemophilia). Furthermore, an increase in thrombin generation is associated with a higher

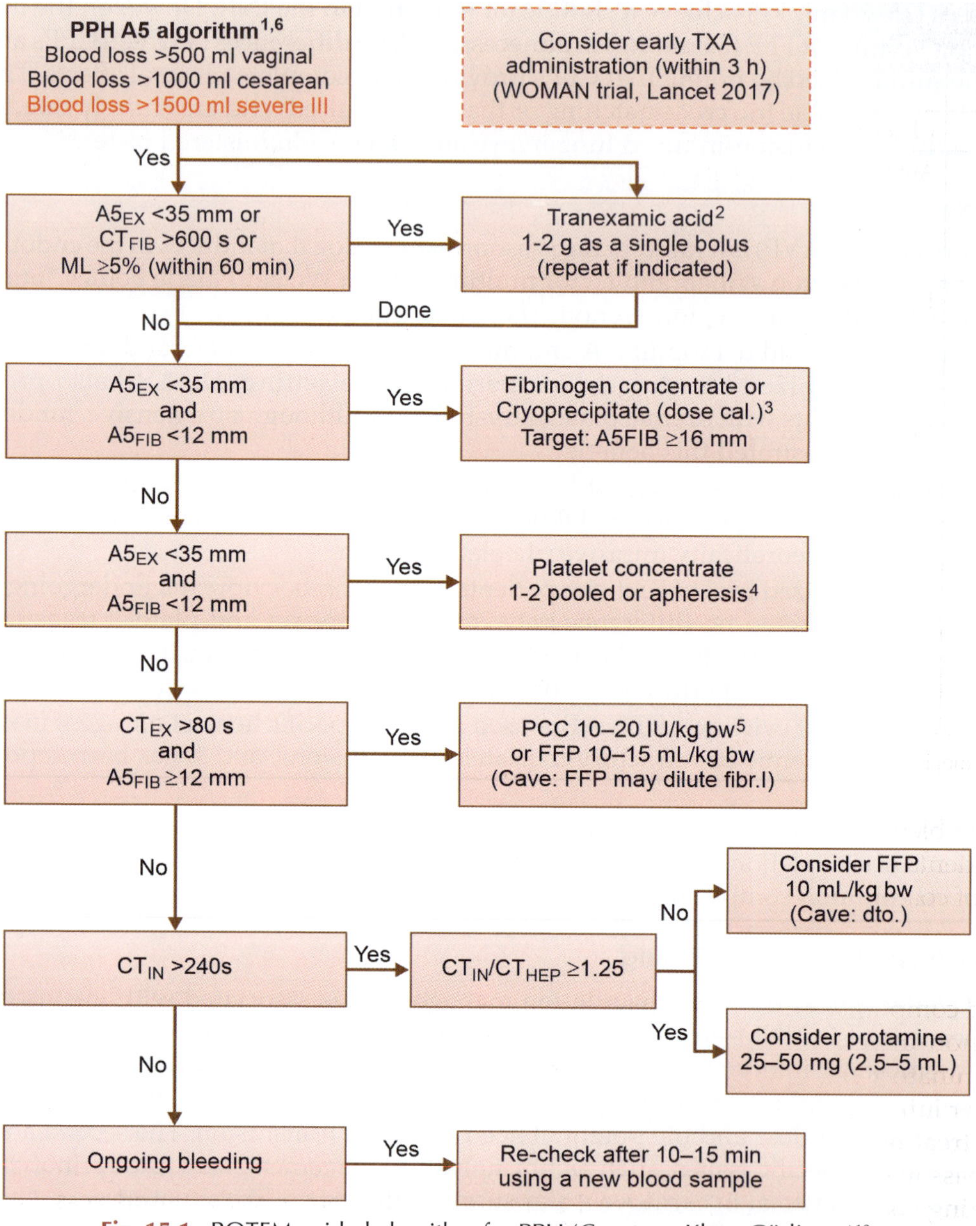

Fig. 15.1: ROTEM guided algorithm for PPH (*Courtesy*: Klaus Görlinger)[12]

risk of thromboembolic complications than substituting substrates, particularly fibrinogen (Fig. 15.1).[10–12]

Treat Basic Conditions

The lethal triad in bleeding patients is coagulopathy, acidosis, and hypothermia. Prevention and treatment include maintaining an objective of treatment of this with the following goals: Temp. > 35°C; pH > 7.2; Cai++ > 1 mmol/L Hb > 7 g/dL. Also, consider early vasopressors to maintain perfusion while maintaining permissive hypotension until a surgical or radiological hemostasis procedure is conducted. ICU starts treatment after the intervention

Table 15.1: Evidence-based algorithms for ROTEM (A5)-guided bleeding management in adult liver transplantation[12]

Step		*Explanation*
1	Check basic conditions	Temp. > 35°C; pH > 7.3; Cai 2+ > 1 mmol/L; Hb ≥ 7 g/dl.
2	Antifibrinolytic therapy	FIB_{CT} > 600 s represents a flat line in FIBTEM. [hyperfibrinolysis increase mortality in PPH]; Tranexamic acid should be administered as first-line treatment without waiting for ROTEM results, according to WOMAN trial.
3	Fibrinogen dose calculation	Fibrinogen dose (g) = targeted increase in A5FIB (mm) × body weight (kg)/160. The correction factor (140–160 mm kg/g) depends on the plasma volume. 10 U Cryoprecipitate ≈2 g fibrinogen concentrate.
4	Platelet concentrate transfusion	Platelet transfusion once fibrinogen is corrected or severe bleeding is developed.
5	Protamine	Endogenous heparin is self-limiting and does not require reversal by Protamine. Consider protamine administration in severe bleeding.
6	Simultaneous interventions	Only in severe bleeding, consider a maximum of three interventions simultaneously. In moderate bleeding, consider a maximum of two interventions simultaneously. There was only one intervention simultaneously (in the second or later analysis and mild to moderate bleeding).

Hb, Hemoglobin; FIB, Fibtem; U, Units; mm, millimeter; kg, kilogram; g, gram.

to stop bleeding, so it is essential to avoid over-transfusion and always consider previous treatments and POC viscoelastic testing in case of persistent bleeding to guide treatment in case of coagulopathy.[12–19]

EVIDENCE CONTOUR

Blood components are high-value resources; however, their use is a risk factor for infectious and non-infectious complications (TRALI, TACO, TRIM), development of a systemic inflammatory response, multiple organ failure, and death.[12] A liberal transfusion policy can further introduce risk to an already compromised patient. Blood is thinned by intravenous fluid treatment, decreasing the concentration of blood cells, platelets, and clotting factors. A decrease in erythrocyte cells causes anemia with decreased O_2 transport capacity, indirectly affecting coagulation. Red cells tend to remain in the center of the blood vessel and push platelets to the periphery near the endothelium.[12] The primary activation of coagulation is caused by the interaction between platelets and this endothelium, and the decrease in hematocrit may cause platelet dysfunction and thrombocytopenia. Transfusion Related Immunomodulation (TRIM) is a non-measurable complication associated with increased mortality, increased multiorgan dysfunction associated with transfusion, increased risk of health-related infection, wound dehiscence, reintervention, ICU and hospital increased length of stay, acute kidney injury among others. Because hemorrhage involves the loss of whole blood, the hemostatic components of blood will inevitably be reduced during active bleeding. Consequently, the hemostatic ability will be reduced in cases of severe bleeding due to consumption; this occurs with an open placental bed on the endometrial surface. Excessive consumption of these factors is then observed in pathological situations such as disseminated intravascular coagulation, placental abruption, retained dead fetus, amniotic fluid embolism, and hemorrhagic shock. These conditions are usually accompanied by excessive hyperfibrinolysis. During fibrinolysis, the clot dissolves prematurely, and in the worst scenario, it will dissolve before the fibrin framework generates adequate hemostasis.[12]

For the last 15 years, a new management concept called "Patient Blood Management" has been a revolutionary approach defined as a "patient-centered, systematic, evidence-based approach to improve patient outcomes by managing and preserving a patient's blood while promoting patient safety and empowerment".."[13]

This approach is a bundle of care that treats risk factors for bleeding and transfusion from a holistic perspective with three pillars of care. 1st pillar is to optimize erythropoiesis, 2nd pillar is coagulation management and bleeding treatment, and the 3rd pillar is to optimize and harness anemia tolerance. This concept of treatment is now endorsed by the World Health Organization (WHO), which in 2021 published the urgent need to implement PBM.[14] However, the bleeding scenario is still challenging, and despite international efforts to try standardized treatment, we still have a long journey ahead to do so.

Lessons learned from the second pillar of PBM in bleeding scenarios

1. Stop the source of bleeding and blood loss
2. Use a restrictive transfusion approach
3. Stop preventive transfusion; it just does not work, and it is essential to understand that.
4. When available viscoelastic testing and goal-directed coagulation therapy should be used.
5. Always create individualized bleeding algorithms and try to keep the approach treat first what kills first (in different bleeding scenarios, stop fibrinolysis or fibrinolysis risk, give clotting strength with fibrinogen and platelets, help trombone generation with PCC preferably if not FFP and finally understand that coagulation is as dynamic as hemodynamics or ventilatory treatments so constantly re-evaluate. Moreover, algorithm treatment should be stopped as soon as the bleeding stops.[12–19]

With these components of the 2nd and 3rd pillars of PBM, it is expected to have better outcomes for patients and excellent economic value by reducing complications, length of stay, and transfusion-related costs, in the management of the patients.[15–18]

REFERENCES

1. Kozek-Langenecker SA, Ahmed AB, Afshari A, Albaladejo P, Aldecoa C, Barauskas G, et al. Management of severe perioperative bleeding: guidelines from the European Society of Anaesthesiology: First update 2016. Eur J Anaesthesiol. 2017;34(6):332–395.
2. Spahn DR, Bouillon B, Cerny V, Coats TJ, Duranteau J, Fernández-Mondéjar E, Filipescu D, Hunt BJ, Komadina R, Nardi G, Neugebauer E, Ozier Y, Riddez L, Schultz A, Vincent JL, Rossaint R. Management of bleeding and coagulopathy following major trauma: an updated European guideline. Crit Care. 2013 Apr 19;17(2):R76.
3. Rossaint R, Bouillon B, Cerny V, Coats TJ, Duranteau J, Fernández-Mondéjar E, Filipescu D, Hunt BJ, Komadina R, Maegele M, Nardi G, Neugebauer E, Ozier Y, Riddez L, Schultz A, Vincent JL, Spahn DR., STOP Bleeding Campaign. The STOP the Bleeding Campaign. Crit Care. 2013 Apr 26;17(2):136.
4. Donley ER, Loyd JW. Hemorrhage Control. [Updated 2022 Jul 19]. In: StatPearls [Internet]. Treasure Island (FL): StatPearls Publishing; 2022 Jan.
5. Colin-Bracamontes I, Pérez-Calatayud ÁA, Carrillo-Esper R, Rodríguez-Ayala E, Padilla-Molina M, Posadas-Nava A, Olvera-Vázquez S, Hernández-Salgado L. Observational Safety Study of Clottafact® Fibrinogen Concentrate: Real-World Data in Mexico. Clin Drug Investig. 2020;40(5):485–491.

6. Abuelkasem E, Hasan S, Mazzeffi MA, Planinsic RM, Sakai T, Tanaka KA. Reduced requirement for prothrombin complex concentrate for the restoration of thrombin generation in plasma from liver transplant recipients. Anesth Analg 2017; 125: 609–15.
7. Refaai MA, Goldstein JN, Lee ML, Durn BL, Milling TJ Jr, Sarode R. Increased risk of volume overload with plasma compared with four factor prothrombin complex concentrate for urgent vitamin K antagonist reversal. Transfusion 2015; 55: 2722–9.
8. Sarode R, Milling TJ Jr, Refaai MA, Mangione A, Schneider A, Durn BL, et al. Efficacy and safety of a 4-factor prothrombin complex concentrate in patients on vitamin K antagonists presenting with major bleeding: a randomized, plasma-controlled, phase IIIb study. Circulation 2013; 128: 1234–43.
9. Nagrebetsky A, Al-Samkari H, Davis NM, Kuter DJ, Wiener-Kronish JP. Perioperative thrombocytopenia: evidence, evaluation, and emerging therapies. Br J Anaesth. 2019;122(1):19–31.
10. Görlinger K, Dirkmann D, Solomon C, Hanke A. Fast interpretation of thromboelastometry in non-cardiac surgery: reliability in patients with hypo-, normo-, and hypercoagulability. British Journal of Anaesthesia 2013;110(2): 220–230.
11. Stettler G, Moore E, Nunns G,Chandler J, Peltz E, Silliman C, et al. Rotational Thromboelastometry thresholds for patients at risk for massive transfusión. Journal of Surgical Research. 2018;228:154–159.
12. Görlinger K, Pérez-Ferrer A, Dirkmann D, Saner F, Maegele M, Calatayud ÁAP, Kim TY. The role of evidence-based algorithms for rotational thromboelastometry-guided bleeding management. Korean J Anesthesiol. 2019;72(4):297–322.
13. Shander A, Hardy JF, Ozawa S, Farmer SL, Hofmann A, Frank SM, Kor DJ, Faraoni D, Freedman J; Collaborators. A Global Definition of Patient Blood Management. Anesth Analg. 2022;135(3):476–488.
14. World Health Organization. (2021). The urgent need to implement patient blood management: policy brief. World Health Organization. https://apps.who.int/iris/handle/10665/346655.
15. Shander A, Goobie SM, Warner MA, Aapro M, Bisbe E, Perez-Calatayud AA, et al.; International Foundation of Patient Blood Management (IFPBM) and Society for the Advancement of Blood Management (SABM) Work Group. Essential Role of Patient Blood Management in a Pandemic: A Call for Action. Anesth Analg. 2020;131(1):74–85.
16. Hofmann A, Spahn DR, Holtorf AP; PBM Implementation Group. Making patient blood management the new norm(al) as experienced by implementors in diverse countries. BMC Health Serv Res. 2021 Jul;21(1):634.
17. Hofmann A, Shander A, Blumberg N, Hamdorf JM, Isbister JP, Gross I. Patient Blood Management: Improving Outcomes for Millions While Saving Billions. What Is Holding It Up? Anesth Analg. 2022 Sep;135(3):511–523.
18. Muñoz M, Stensballe J, Ducloy-Bouthors AS, Bonnet MP, De Robertis E, Fornet I, Goffinet F, Hofer S, Holzgreve W, Manrique S, Nizard J, Christory F, Samama CM, Hardy JF. Patient blood management in obstetrics: prevention and treatment of postpartum haemorrhage. A NATA consensus statement. Blood Transfus. 2019;17(2):112–136.
19. Manejo hemático del paciente. Guía de Práctica Clínica: Evidencias y Recomendaciones. México, CENETEC; 2020 [fecha de consulta]. Disponible en: http://www.cenetec- difusion.com/CMGPC/GPC-SS-830-20/ER.pdf
20. Borowko R, Vignon PO, Lutz N, Maillot A, Lefort H. La triade létale de l'hémorragie [The lethal triad of hemorrhage]. Rev Infirm. 2021 Aug-Sep;70(273):16–18.

CHAPTER

16

Management of "Acute Coronary Syndrome": A Case Based Approach

Sandeep Kantor, Juhi Chandwani, Huda Al Khalili

CASE

A 60-year-old gentleman came to ER with crushing chest pain radiating to his jaw and left arm, with difficulty in breathing and altered sensorium. He was immediately given 800 µg of glyceryl trinitrate (GTN) spray, and aspirin 300 mg orally.

On arrival, patient was in a peri-arrest state. He was still complaining of central chest pain and was diaphoretic. He was desaturating to 84% on non-rebreathing mask, and his blood gas (arterial) revealed mixed respiratory and metabolic acidosis. His chest X-ray and ECG was unremarkable. Cardiac markers were not elevated. A bedside echocardiogram revealed left ventricular global hypokinesia. The bystanders gave a history that patient smoked at least 20 cigarettes daily (38 packs per year), but there were no other cardiac risk factors. Despite unremarkable ECG, cardiac enzymes and chest X-ray, diagnosis of acute coronary syndrome (ACS) was made in view of echo-cardiographic features.

What is Appropriate Management for this Patient?

Ans: Cardiac catheterization (CAG) for urgent percutaneous coronary intervention in view of severe left ventricular dysfunction. CAG showed stenosis of the left main stem coronary artery, which was stented uneventfully, and patient recovered without any complications.

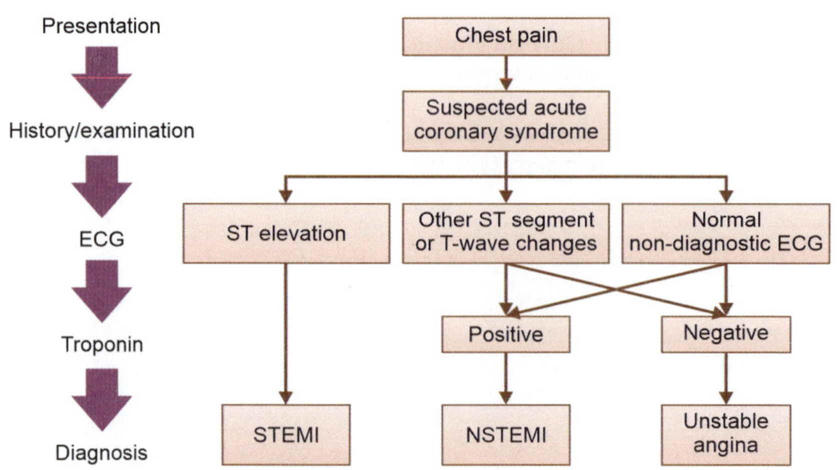

Fig. 16.1: The classification of acute coronary syndrome

The Burden of Acute Coronary Syndrome and Principles of Management

Although significant advances have been made in the management of ACS, cardiovascular disease is the leading cause of mortality worldwide mainly due to ischaemic heart disease.[1] Modern management strategies have enabled early detection, appropriate triaging and improved outcome.

Diagnosis: ACS diagnosis is based on triad of clinical manifestations, ECG findings, and biochemical markers of myocardial damage. Management of a patient with ACS is based on ST-segment evaluation on ECG. ST segment elevation MI (STEMI) are easier to diagnose with 12-lead ECG. NSTE (non-ST-elevation)-ACS which includes unstable angina and NSTEMI, requires supportive evidence with rising troponins (high sensitive, hsTn) assays, serial ECGs, echocardiography or cardiac MRI, which may reveal regional wall motion abnormalities (RWMA) in patients presenting with clinical features of acute coronary syndromes.

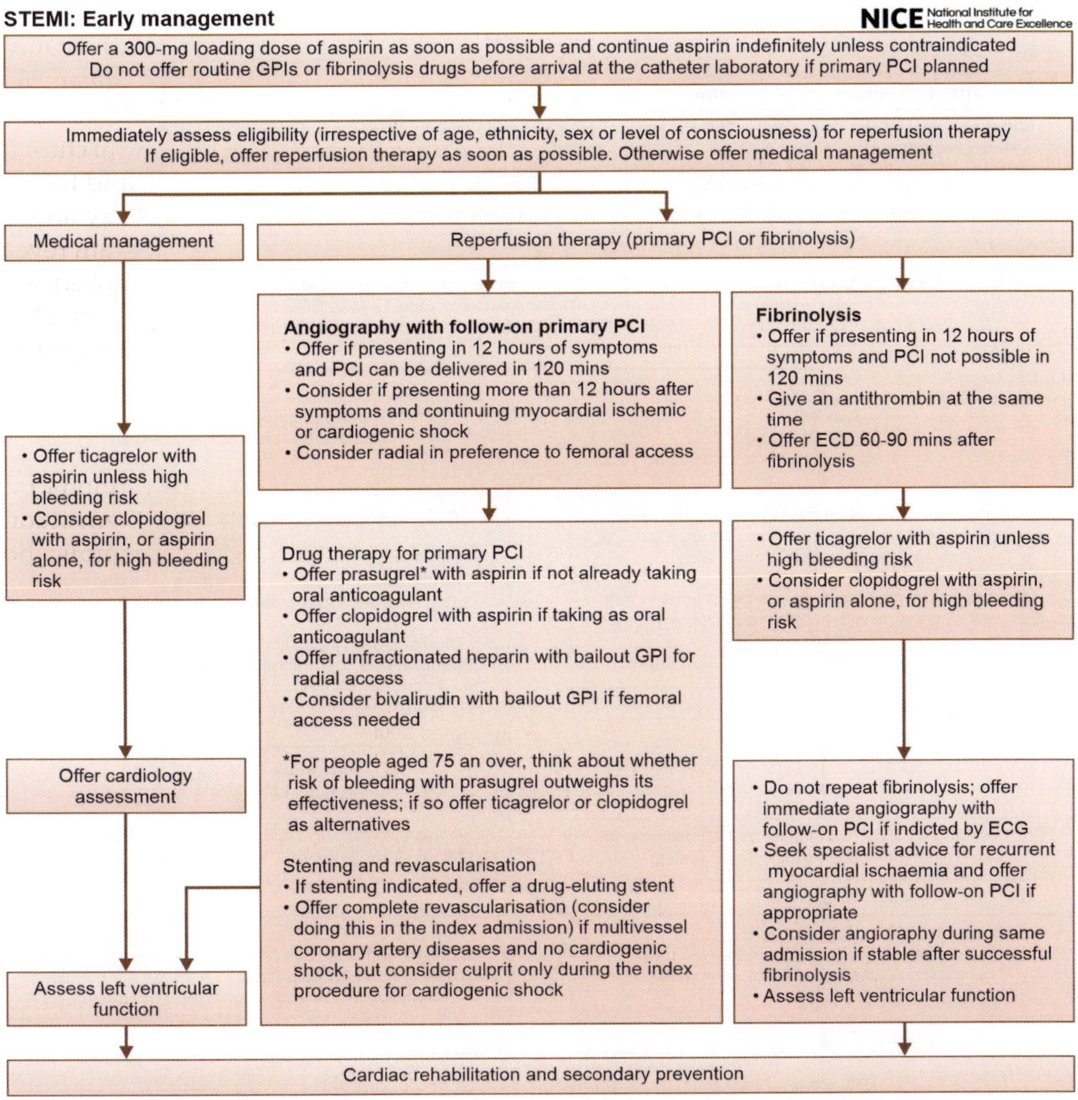

Fig. 16.2: Standard ST elevation myocardial infarction management

We have covered evidence from all reputed societies which have updated their recommendations on management of ACS (STEMI and NSTEMI) which include NICE (National Institute of Health & Care Excellence),[2] American College of Cardiology 3 in conjunction with American Heart Association (AHA/ACC) and the European Society of Cardiology (ESC).[4,5,6,7] With the Covid-19 pandemic, almost all the associations, made significant changes to their approach to patients with acute coronary syndrome.

STEMI—Early Assessment and Management[7,8,9,10,11]

- All patients with STEMI should get 300 mg aspirin immediately in absence of any allergy.
- A meticulous assessment in ACS patients with STEMI for coronary reperfusion strategy either with primary PCI or fibrinolysis should be made.
- All patients with STEMI, irrespective of level of consciousness post-arrest, merit coronary angiography (with follow-on primary PCI if indicated).

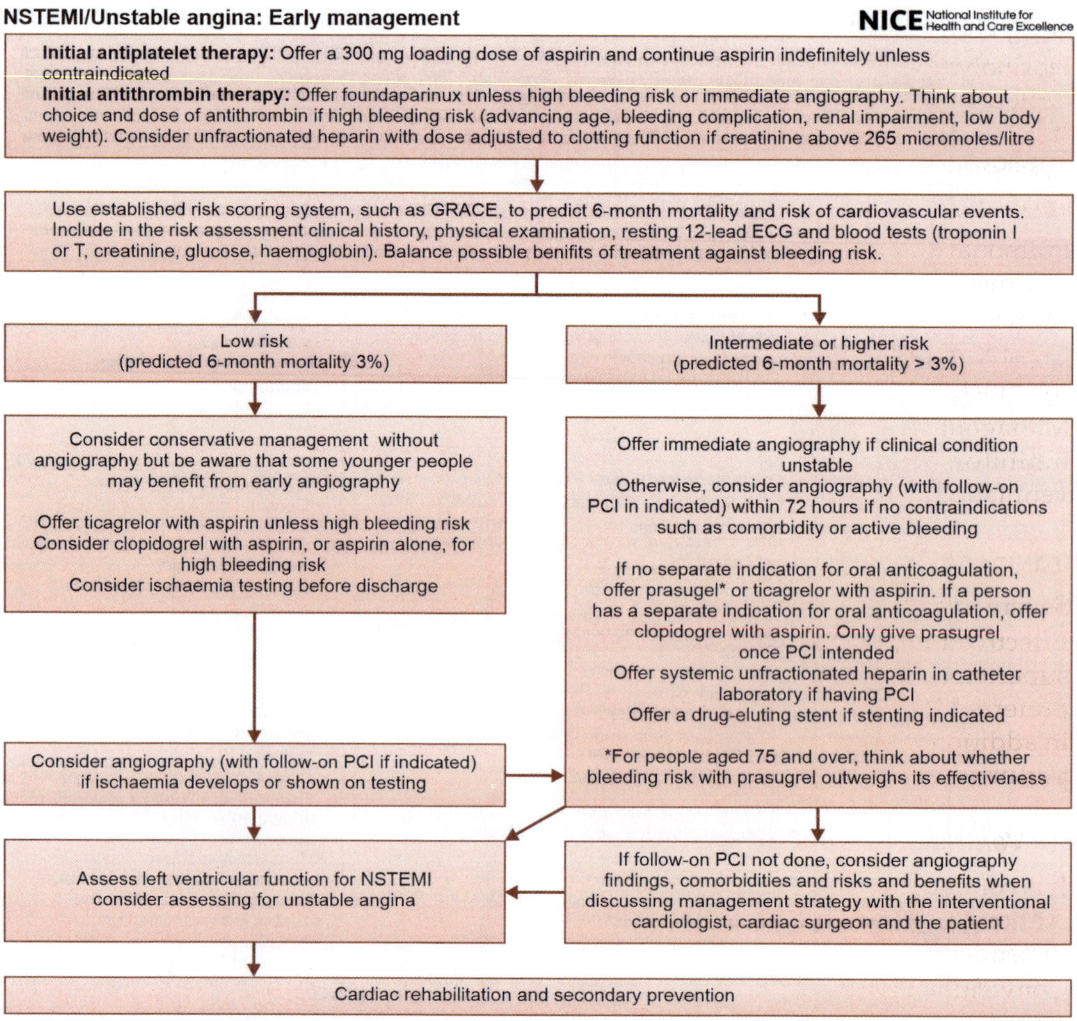

Fig. 16.3: Non-ST-elevation of myocardial infarction management

- Urgent CAG with +/– PCI is recommended in patients arriving within 12 hours of symptom onset. Patients presenting after 12 hours with evidence of ongoing myocardial ischemia and those presenting with cardiogenic shock, should also undergo coronary angiography.
- Glycoprotein IIb/IIIa inhibitors or fibrinolytic agents should be avoided in patients with acute STEMI going for primary PCI.
- Dual antiplatelet therapy (DAPT) with aspirin and prasugrel should be considered for all irrespective of PCI. In patients taking oral anticoagulants, aged above 75 years or having high bleeding risk, clopidogrel or ticagrelor is offered.
- Unfractionated heparin and glycoprotein IIb/IIIa with DAPT is anticoagulation of choice when radial access is used for PCI. Femoral access PCI, requires bivalirudin instead of heparin.
- Aspiration of thrombus is performed but not a routine.
- Only culprit vessel revascularization is the treatment of choice for patients with cardiogenic shock, whereas in patients without cardiogenic shock with multivessel coronary artery disease complete revascularization should be done.
- Drug-eluting stent is preferred over plain metal stents as they have less mortality.
- Fibrinolysis in those patients where primary PCI cannot be done should be given within 12 hours of symptoms.

Complications of STEMI

Pulmonary Edema

- Pulmonary edema develops due to left ventricular failure, and it can present as increased shortness of breath, hypoxia related tachycardia, third heart sound and basal rales. Other causes of heart failure such as rhythm and valvular abnormality should be ruled out.
- Chest X-ray would show lung congestion and echocardiography will reveal left ventricular dysfunction in the form of akinesia or reduced ejection fraction.
- Management includes decongestion with diuretics, intravenous nitrates, with ACE inhibitors. In some individuals respiratory support with noninvasive or invasive ventilation may be needed. Reperfusion therapy remains the mainstay of treatment.

Cardiogenic Shock

- Severe myocardial dysfunction in patients with STEMI can lead to cardiogenic shock.
- Effective myocardial reperfusion therapy in form of PCI is preferred treatment and is superior to thrombolysis. Inotropes (preferably Noradrenaline +/– Dobutamine) are preferred in patients with cardiogenic shock, and sometimes intra-aortic balloon pump in addition to vasoactive drugs may be required where there is reduced cerebral or renal perfusion.

Right Ventricular Dysfunction

- It is commonly seen with inferior wall infarction. Isolated cases of RV dysfunction is rare. Although pulmonary edema is absent but patients will present with hypotension and distended neck veins.
- Conventional left-sided ECG may not reveal RV dysfunction. If suspected right-sided ECG recording (V4R) should be done which is highly sensitive and specific for inferior infarction.

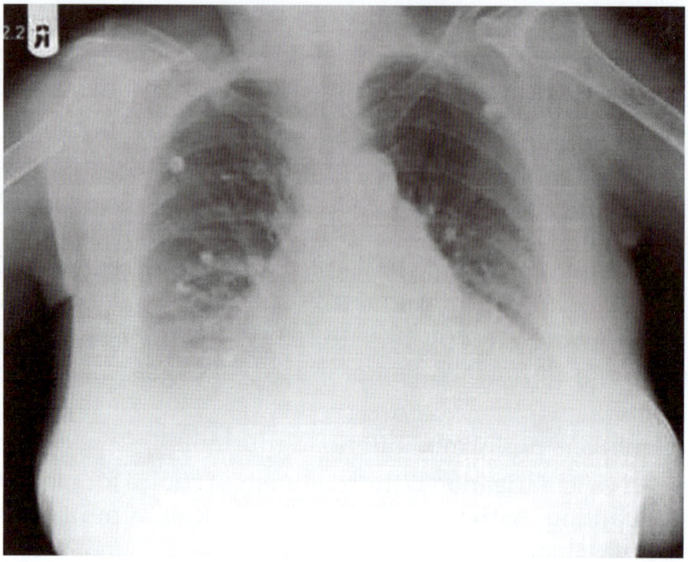

Fig. 16.4

- Echocardiography will further support diagnosis and will reveal presence of tricuspid valve incompetence.
- Right ventricular preload should be maintained, if needed with a fluid challenge with close hemodynamic monitoring in these patients, to avoid hypotension which may be aggravated due to nitrates and opiates given as part of STEMI management.
- Reperfusion remains the cornerstone of management to improve the haemodynamic state.

All patients of before discharge should have left ventricular assessment done, for treatment optimization.

Management of NSTEMI and Unstable Angina[12]

- A single loading dose of 300 mg aspirin should be offered to all patients to be continued indefinitely in patients with NSTEMI/unstable angina, in absence of any allergy or other contraindication.
- Anticoagulant therapy should be chosen carefully in patients with high bleeding risk especially in old age, and low body weight and renal impairment. Those with renal impairment without any bleeding risk, Fondaparinux or unfractionated heparin should be offered with dose adjustment unless patient is proceeding for immediate coronary angioplasty.
- All patients diagnosed with unstable angina or NSTEMI presenting with chest pain warrant dual antiplatelet therapy.

Risk Assessment

- Risk assessment of future major adverse cardiovascular events is mandated for all ACS including NSTEMI after immediate management with drugs. This is done using GRACE score which predicts six-month mortality and helps in planning further care. (Figs 16.5a and b:[12] BMJ visual summary)
- NICE gives recommendations for PCI versus conservative management based on predicted risk of cardiovascular events and 6 months mortality, as shown in Tables 16.1 and 16.2.[12]

Table 16.1: Categorizing risk of future adverse cardiovascular events	
Predicted 6-month mortality	***Risk of future adverse cardiovascular events***
1.5% or below	Lowest
>1.5% to 3.0%	Low
>3.0% to 6.0%	Intermediate
>6.0% to 9.0%	High
Over 9.0%	Highest

*The guideline is available from the NICE website (https://www.nice.org.uk/guidance/ng185)
Categories of risk are derived from the Myocardial Ischemia National Audit Project (MINAP) database.

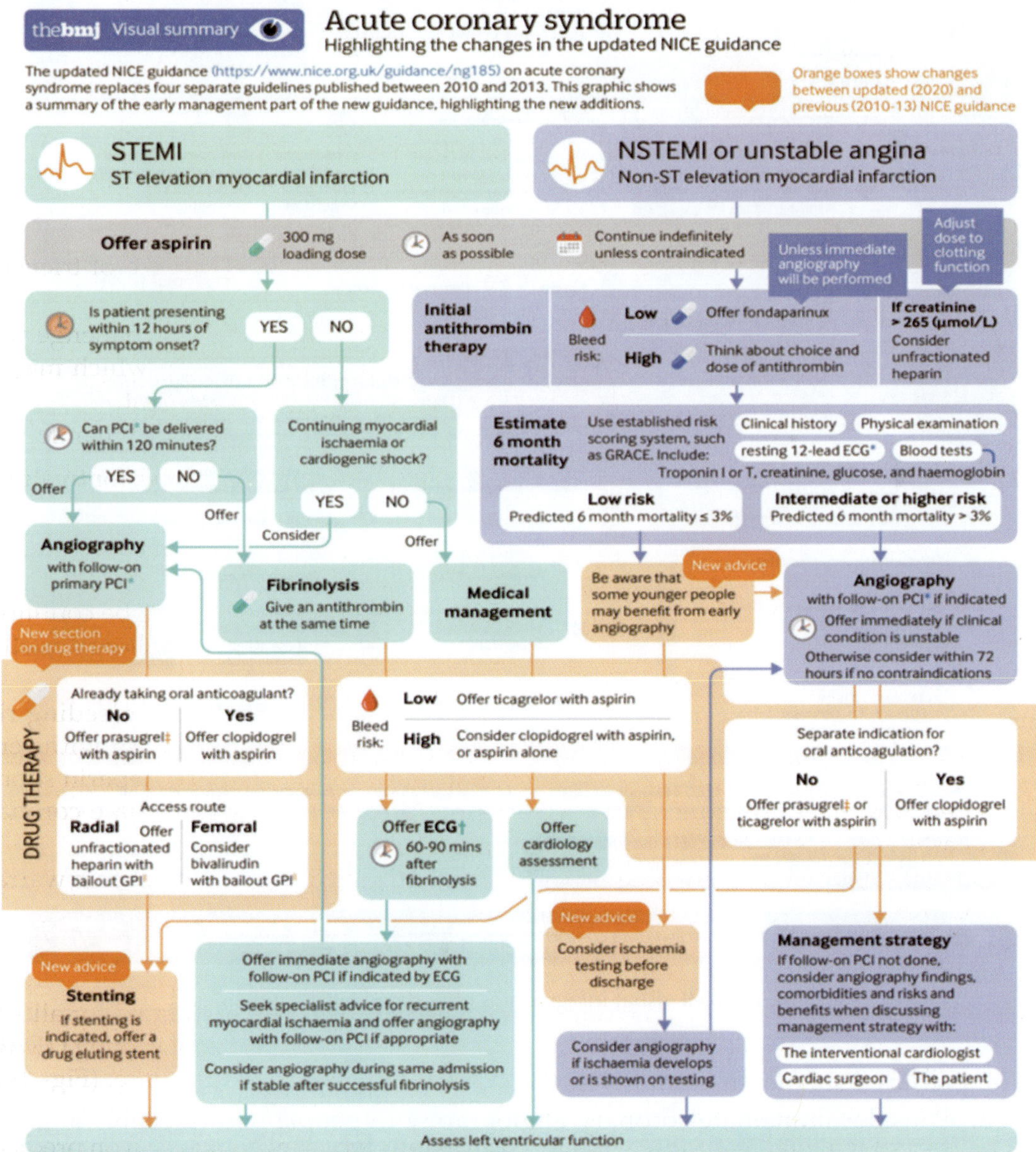

Fig. 16.5a: BMJ visual infographics of updated NICE guidelines

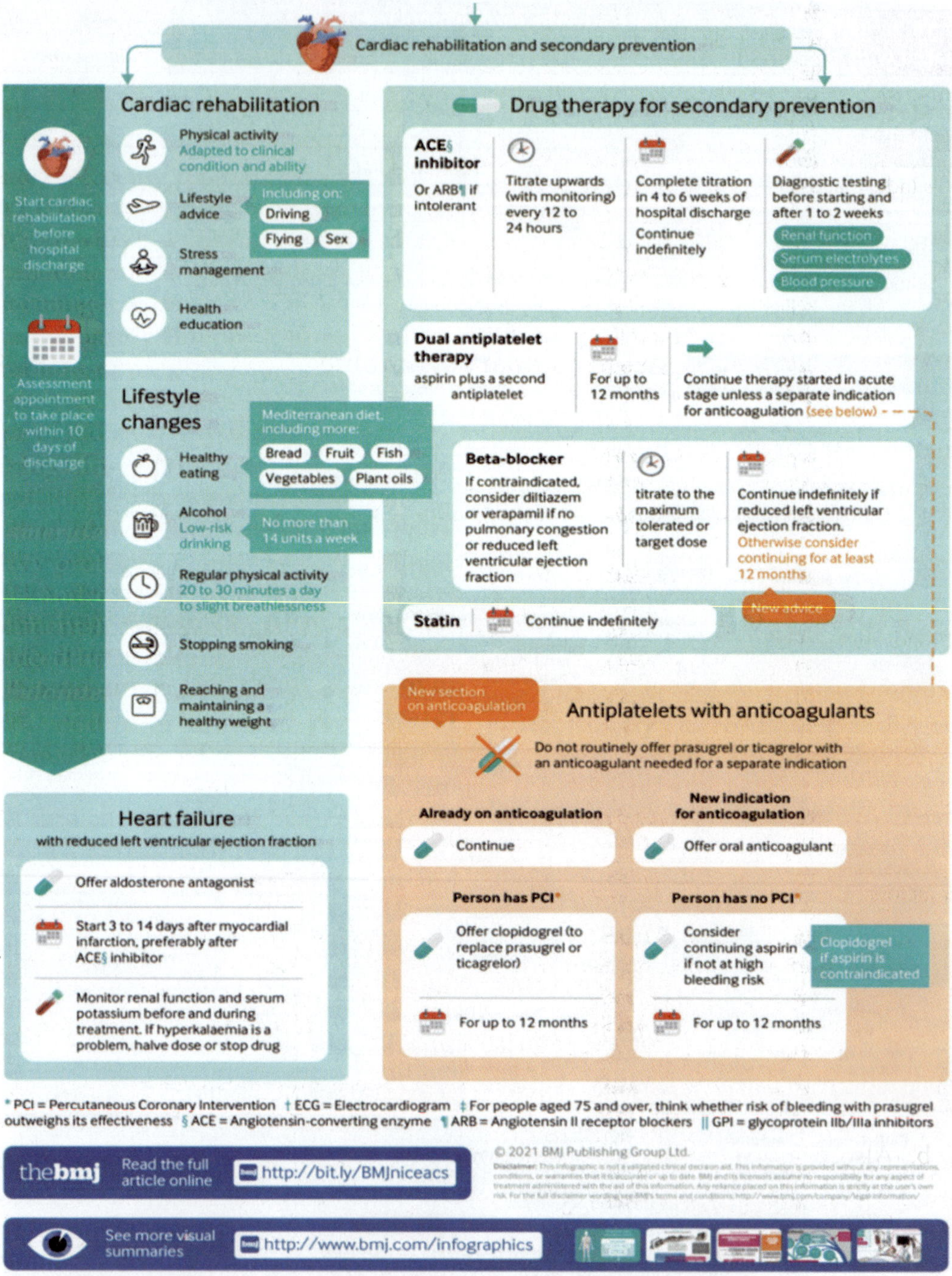

Fig. 16.5b: BMJ visual infographics of updated NICE guidelines

1. If predicted six-month mortality ≤3.0%
   a. Consider immediate coronary angiography to people with unstable angina or NSTEMI if their clinical condition is unstable or if their ischemia symptoms return subsequently as demonstrated by ischemia testing.

Table 16.2: Benefits and risks of early invasive treatment (coronary angiography with PCI if needed) compared with conservative management for people with unstable angina or NSTEMI

Benefits/risks/other factors	*Coronary angiography and possible percutaneous coronary intervention (PCI) within 72 hours*	*Conservative management with later coronary angiography if problems continue or develop*
Benefits (advantages)	Reduced deaths from all causes at 6 to 12 months and at 2 years. Reduced deaths from heart problems at 1 and 2 years. Reduced incidence of myocardial infarction (MI) at 30 days, 6 to 12 months and 2 years. Reduced incidence of stroke at 1 year, particularly in people at high risk of future adverse events. Reduced readmission to hospital and difficult-to-treat angina in the medium term, particularly in people at high risk of future adverse events. Psychological benefits—people are not anxious about delaying angiography.	Avoid the immediate risks of invasive treatment, including: • Death within 4 months related to the procedure from causes other than MI • Procedure-related MI • Major bleeding in hospital and up to 2 years after the procedure. These are particularly relevant for people at low risk of future adverse events. Psychological benefits—people are not anxious about having an invasive procedure.
Risk (disadvantages)	Increased risk of death during first 4 months, particularly for people at low risk of future adverse events Risk of procedure-related MI Increased risk of major bleeding during index admission at 30 days and 2 years. Emergency treatment leaves a little time for shared decision making.	Increased risk of MI after 6 months. Increased risk of stroke at 1 year, particularly in people at high risk of future adverse events. Psychological factors—people may be anxious about delaying angiography.
Other factors	Recent advances in PCI might increase early benefit, particularly reducing bleeding. Coronary angiography within 72 hours ensures speedy intervention while allowing time for correct diagnosis, identifying other treatment and treating conditions	

b. Also, consider early coronary angiography for some younger people with low risk scores for mortality at 6 months if they are at high risk of adverse cardiovascular events.

c. Do not offer dual anti-platelet therapy to people with chest pain before a diagnosis of unstable angina or NSTEMI is made.

2. All risk and benefits of various options should be explained to the patient so as to obtain an informed consent.
3. If the mortality is expected to be more than 3%
   a. Consider coronary angiography (with follow-on PCI if indicated) within 72 hours of first admission for people with unstable angina or NSTEMI if there is no contraindications to angiography (such as active bleeding or comorbidity).

Hyperglycemia in Acute Coronary Syndromes[13]

Hyperglycemia needs to be controlled post-ACS for up to 48 hours, with insulin infusion if required to maintain blood glucose levels below 11 mmol/L. Following ACS, there is increased risk of developing type 2 diabetes and hence patients require regular assessment with lifestyle changes.

Secondary Prevention[14]

ACE inhibitors, calcium channel blockers and/or aldosterone antagonist should be offered to all patients post-MI for secondary prevention.

All patients need to continue DAPT for 12 months unless contraindicated.

If anticoagulation needs to be started for new indication following PCI, clopidogrel should replace prasugrel or ticagrelor as they are contraindicated in such patients.

Beta-blocker may be given for maximum 12 months after an MI in patients without evidence of low ejection fraction.

Hypertension management is of paramount importance in all patients with MI.

Cardiac Rehabilitation after an MI[15]

- Appropriate rehabilitation program after MI should be offered to everyone.
- The programs should be holistic involving family and include health education, stress management, lifestyle modification including psychological health.
- Sexual activity can be resumed after four weeks in those with an uneventful recovery.
- Cardiac rehabilitation requires diet modification, moderate alcohol consumption, regular exercise, physical activity, smoking cessation and weight control.

Evidence Contour

Over the years multiple trials have been done to find effective therapy for ACS. Some of the major trials have given robust evidence of effective and safe treatment like:
- Antiplatelet therapy is the mainstay of treatment with aspirin and clopidogrel shown to improve mortality.
- Newer P2Y12 inhibitors improve mortality further but possibly not those who are conservatively managed.
- Along with that anti-thrombotic therapy is beneficial and unfractionated heparin appears more efficacious.
- PCI for STEMI is superior to thrombolysis, even when performed routinely after thrombolysis. PCI is also beneficial in NSTEMI patients.
- Secondary prevention is equally important with statins having shown to reduce recurrent cardiovascular events along with ACE inhibitors and beta blockers as indicated.

However, in spite of these trials, controversies remain regarding safety and efficacy of pharmacological treatment, which the practising clinician needs to address and modify as per individual patient needs.[16]

Antiplatelet Therapy

Clopidogrel in unstable angina to prevent Recurrent ischemic Events (CURE) trial, established evidence for DAPT which is treating all ACS patients with 300 mg of clopidogrel after loading with 300 mg to aspirin in ACS, irrespective PCI.[17] However, OASIS 7 trial demonstrated that this increased the risk of major bleeds by 24% especially in patients undergoing PCI for ACS.[18]

Recent evidence supports aspirin bolus of 300 mg for ACS patients followed by maintenance low dose of 75 mg. Initiation of the P2Y12 inhibitor (e.g. Clopidogrel) remains a subject of much controversy. None of the major prospective randomized trials gave a definitive answer as to the optimal time for loading with clopidogrel or ticagrelor.[19]

Another debating point is the duration of DAPT. Individualized treatment decisions with DAPT agents require tools like DAPT score which will help in balancing risk with ischemia prevention in patients with ACS. High GI bleeding risk requires early cessation of aspirin after 3 months. Most trials have shown SAPT (single antiplatelet therapy) is not to be inferior to dual therapy.[20]

Clopidogrel is a prodrug, and it requires biotransformation by hepatic CYP450 enzyme. This is influenced by CYP2C19 locus loss of function carriers in some patients with ACS on clopidogrel. As a result they become prone to major adverse cardiovascular events (MACE). Still, genotype and platelet function directed therapy has not been well accepted. The decision is always based on clinical judgement.

Parenteral Anticoagulants

Unfractionated heparin, enoxaparin and fondaparinux are choice agents in all patient requiring reperfusion therapy. Heparin is preferred agent being cost effective, safer compared to Bivalirudin or Glycoprotein IIb/IIIa inhibitors in renal patients and in addition and its effect being easily reversible with protamine. European guidelines use fondaparinux as first-line anticoagulant agent in ischemia-guided strategies, whereas the AHA/ACC makes no preference. Most places, parenteral anticoagulation is typically a decision between heparin and Glycoprotein IIb/IIIa inhibitors versus bivalirudin if proceeding to PCI.[21]

Triple Therapy Controversy

Anticoagulation is indicated for atrial fibrillation which may develop in 8–10% of ACS patients requiring PCI. This combination of DAPT plus an oral anticoagulant enhances bleeding risk in ACS patients. Lower rates of bleeding have been found with Direct-Acting Oral Anticoagulants (DOAC) than vitamin K agonist triple antithrombotic therapy. However, this may lead to increased risk of myocardial infarction and stent thrombosis, but the studies did not reach statistical significance.

2020 European guidelines suggest one week of triple antithrombotic therapy (or until hospital discharge) followed by dual antithrombotic therapy with a DOAC plus P2Y 12 inhibitor (typically clopidogrel) for 1 year, following that only DOAC monotherapy could be given. Bleeding risk should be assessed on the therapy and treatment tailored accordingly.[3]

Drug Related Problems in ACS Management

Clopidogrel remains mainstay of DAPT in ACS patients. Since DAPT may increase risk of gastrointestinal bleeds, proton pump inhibitors like omeprazole or esomeprazole are commonly given. However, this may interact with CYP2C19 mediated conversion of clopidogrel to its active form in the liver, thus contributing to increased risk of MACE. PPIs such as lansoprazole and dexlansoprazole have been found to have less effect, and pantoprazole and rabeprazole do not affect the metabolism of clopidogrel. Hence appropriate PPI should be chosen in patients requiring a combination of clopidogrel and PPI.[22]

Crucial elements of management are secondary preventive strategies in ACS. These measures are strict lipid lowering therapy, neurohormonal agents, and lifestyle changes.

Since adherence to medications is a major issue, patient's need to be counseled appropriately. Clinical pharmacists can play a major role in addressing these issues to manage comorbidities and polypharmacy in these patients.

REFERENCES

1. Global Burden of Disease Collaborators. Global burden of 369 diseases and injuries in 204 countries and territories, 1990–2019 a sysematic analysis for the Global Burden of Disease Study 2019. Lancet 2020. 396: 1204 –42.
2. Acute coronary syndromes. NICE guideline. Published: 18 November 2020. Available at www.nice.org.uk/guidance/ng185
3. Collet JP, Thiele H, Barbato E, Barthelemy O, Bauerachs J, Bhatt DL et al. ESC Scientific Document Group, 2020 ESC Guidelines for the management of acute coronary syndromes in patients presenting without persistent ST-segment elevation: The Task Force for the management of acute coronary syndromes in patients presenting without persistent ST-segment elevation of the European Society of Cardiology (ESC), European Heart Journal, 2021;42(14):1289–1367.
4. O'Gara PT, Kushner FG, Ascheim DD, Casey DE Jr, Chung MK, de Lemos JA et al. 2013 ACCF/AHA guideline for the management of ST-elevation myocardial infarction: a report of the American College of Cardiology Foundation/American Heart Association Task Force on Practice Guidelines. J Am Coll Cardiol. 2013;61(4):e78–e140.
5. Steg PG, James SK, Atar D, Badano LP, et al. ESC guidelines for the management of acute myocardial infarction in patients presenting with ST segment elevation. Eur Heart J. 2012;33(20):2569–619.
6. Busko M. New ESC guideline on acute ST-segment elevation MI. Medscape Medical News. Available at https://www.medscape.com/viewarticle/885509. September 11, 2017; Accessed: August 27, 2018.
7. National Clinical Guideline Centre (UK). Myocardial Infarction with ST-Segment Elevation: The Acute Management of Myocardial Infarction with ST-Segment Elevation [Internet]. London: Royal College of Physicians (UK); 2013 Jul. PMID: 25340241.
8. National Guideline Centre (UK). Evidence review for dual antiplatelet therapy: Acute Coronary Syndromes: Evidence review A. London: National Institute for Health and Care Excellence (NICE); 2020 Nov. PMID: 33301275.
9. Guedeney P, Collet JP. Antithrombotic Therapy in Acute Coronary Syndromes: Current Evidence and Ongoing Issues Regarding Early and Late Management. Thromb Haemost. 2021;121(7):854–866.
10. National Guideline Centre (UK). Evidence review for antithrombin therapy in adults with ST-segment elevation myocardial infarction intended for primary percutaneous coronary intervention: Acute Coronary Syndromes: Evidence review D. London: National Institute for Health and Care Excellence (NICE); 2020 Nov.
11. National Guideline Centre (UK). Evidence review for dual antiplatelet therapy: Acute Coronary Syndromes: Evidence review A. London: National Institute for Health and Care Excellence (NICE); 2020 Nov.
12. Corbett SJ, Ftouh S, Lewis S, Lovibond K; Guideline Committee. Acute coronary syndromes: summary of updated NICE guidance. BMJ. 2021;372:m4760.
13. Angeli F, Reboldi G, Poltronieri C, Lazzari L, Sordi M, Garofoli M et al. Hyperglycemia in acute coronary syndromes: from mechanisms to prognostic implications. Ther Adv Cardiovasc Dis. 2015;9(6):412–24.
14. Hypertension in adults: diagnosis and management. London: National Institute for Health and Care Excellence (NICE); 2022 Mar 18. PMID: 31577399.
15. Chaplin, S. (2021), NICE on the management of acute coronary syndromes. Prescriber, 32: 26–27.
16. Colin T Phillips, Michael C Gavin. Controversies in Antiplatelet and Anticoagulation Therapy in Patients Presenting with Acute Coronary Syndrome, US Cardiology Review 2017;11(2):52–8.
17. Mora S, Ames JM, Manson JE. Low-dose aspirin in the primary prevention of cardiovascular disease: shared decision making in clinical practice. JAMA 2016;316(7):709–10.

18. Mehta SR, Tanguay JF, Eikelboom JW, Jolly SS, Joyner CD, Granger CB et al. CURRENT-OASIS 7 trial investigators. Double-dose versus standard-dose clopidogrel and high-dose versus low-dose aspirin in individuals undergoing percutaneous coronary intervention for acute coronary syndromes (CURRENT-OASIS 7): a randomised factorial trial. Lancet. 2010;376(9748):1233–43.
19. Bergmark BA, Mathenge N, Merlini PA, Lawrence-Wright MB, Giugliano RP. Acute coronary syndromes. Lancet. 2022;399(10332):1347–1358.
20. Yeh RW, Secemsky EA, Kereiakes DJ, Normand SLT, Gerschlik AH, Cohen DJ et al. Development and validation of a prediction rule for benefit and harm of dual antiplatelet therapy beyond 1 year after percutaneous coronary intervention. JAMA 2016;315(16):1735–49.
21. Rodriguez F, Mahaffey KW. Management of patients with NSTEACS: a comparison of the recent AHA/ACC and ESC guidelines. J Am Coll Cardiol 2016;68(3):313–21.
22. Tran AV, Nguyen DT, Tran SK, Vo TH, Nguyen KT, Nguyen PM et al. Drug-Related Problems in Coronary Artery Diseases. In: Murashita, T., editor. Coronary Artery Bypass Grafting [Internet]. London: IntechOpen; 2022.

CHAPTER

17 Management of Pulmonary Embolism: A Case Based Approach

Gentle Sunder Shrestha, Sachit Sharma

CASE DESCRIPTION

A 45-year-male presented to the emergency department with the chief complaints of sudden onset shortness of breath and racing of the heart. He was a known case of hypertension and diabetes. On evaluation in the emergency department, his blood pressure was 80/50 mmHg, heart rate was 140 beats per minute and with temperature of 99 degree Fahrenheit. Chest imaging was performed which revealed regional oligemia in the right upper zone and an enlarged pulmonary artery. Echocardiography revealed left atrial size of 5 cm and severe tricuspid regurgitation. ECG revealed a sinus tachycardia. Subsequently, a CT pulmonary angiogram was performed.

What should be the Approach for Immediate Management of this Patient?

Ans: Volume optimization using normal saline or lactated Ringer's in a volume of around 500 ml administered over 15 to 30 minutes, use of inotropes and vasopressors, preferably norepinephrine or dopamine is the mainstay of treatment for hemodynamic support. Endotracheal intubation need to be considered for respiratory support and in the event of worsening hemodynamic status. Since this patient also shows features of right ventricular failure, administration of thrombolytic agents results in more rapid resolution of pulmonary obstruction and helps in faster achievement of hemodynamic stability. For patients who remain hemodynamically unstable despite thrombolytic therapy and all other supportive measures, mechanical circulatory support using Veno-Arterial ECMO/ECLS can be provided as a rescue therapy for hemodynamic and respiratory support.

PRINCIPLES OF MANAGEMENT

Diagnosis

Several factors need to be considered for diagnosing pulmonary embolism (PE). Clinical presentation is the first among them.

a. *Clinical features*: Chest pain, dyspnea, presyncope or syncope demand a high suspicion of PE. Hemodynamic instability is a less common but an important finding and often indicates central or extensive PE. Hypoxemia and hypocapnia may be often present but does not occur in all patients. Chest X-ray often helps to rule out the differentials of PE. Findings suggestive of right ventricular strain like T wave inversion in precordial leads V_1 and V_4, QR pattern in lead V_1, $S_1Q_3T_3$ pattern, and incomplete or complete right bundle branch block pattern are more commonly seen in cases of severe PE.[1] Furthermore, assessment of the risk factors for VTE is also essential in clinically evaluating the pre-test probability.

b. Clinical (pre-test) probability: Clinical features in conjunction with predisposing factors for PE allow patients with suspected PE to be classified into different categories which correlates with the cases of confirmed PE. This can be performed either clinically or by using various prediction rules. Among the prediction rules, Revised Geneva rule and the Wells rule are most commonly used. Irrespective of the scoring system used, the probability of confirmed PE is around 10% in the low-probability group, 30% in the moderate-probability group, and 65% in the high probability group.[2] The probability of patients with confirmed PE is around 12% in the PE-unlikely category and 30% in the PE-likely category while using the two level classification system.[2]
c. Pulmonary embolism rule out criteria (PERC): To avoid overuse of diagnostic testing for suspected PE, a patient with low clinical probability and fulfilling the PERC rule criteria can be safely excluded. PERC rule comprises of eight clinical variables significantly associated with an absence of PE: age <50 years; pulse <100 beats per minute; SaO_2 >94%; no unilateral leg swelling; no hemoptysis; no recent trauma or surgery; no history of VTE; and no oral hormone use.[3,4]
d. D-dimer: In acute PE, due to activation of coagulation and fibrinolysis together, D-dimer levels can be raised. The diagnostic accuracy of ELISA derived D-dimer assays to rule out PE is >= 95% in patients with low or intermediate probability PE. The negative predictive value of D-dimer is high rendering this test useful to exclude PE if the value is within normal range. The low positive predictive value makes the test less useful to diagnose PE if the value is high (Flowchart 17.1).
e. CT pulmonary angiogram (CTPA): Multidetector CTPA allows proper visualization of the pulmonary vasculature up to the subsegmental level. Rather than using it as a standalone test, the predictive value can be enhanced if this test is combined with clinical probability testing. A negative CTPA had a high negative predictive value for PE in patients with low or intermediate clinical probability for PE (96 and 89%, respectively). However, if the pre-test probability is high, the negative predictive value is only 60%. In contrary, in patients with intermediate or high clinical probability, the positive predictive value of a positive CTPA is high (92–96%). Of note, in patients with a low pre-test likelihood of PE, the incidence of PE is lower (around 58%).[5] Further testing need to be considered if there is disparity between clinical judgement and the CTPA result (Flowchart 17.2).
f. Pulmonary angiography: Echocardiography—acute PE can cause changes in the RV size and function. However, a negative echocardiography result has a negative predictive value of around 40–50% and should not be used to exclude PE.[6] RV dilation can be found in ≥ 25% of patients with PE. Echocardiographic finding of decreased pulmonary ejection acceleration time (less than 60 ms) in conjunction with a lower peak systolic tricuspid valve gradient of less than 60 mmHg ('60/'60 sign) or diminished contractility of RV free wall have a high positive predictive value in patients with PE.[7] Echocardiography may also reveal decreased tricuspid annular plane systolic excursion (TAPSE).[8] The utility of echocardiography as a diagnostic modality is more in hemodynamically unstable patients with suspected PE in whom a normal echocardiography practically excludes PE as the cause of hemodynamic instability. On the other hand, in a patient with suspected PE and hemodynamic instable, echocardiographic features of RV pressure overload like presence of right heart thrombi, 60/60 sign, or McConnell sign would warrant emergency reperfusion therapy, provided urgent CT angiography is not feasible and if the patient does not have other obvious causes for RV pressure overload.[9] It is not mandatory to perform echocardiography in hemodynamically stable patients.[6]

Flowchart 17.1: Algorithm for diagnosis of PE in patients without hemodynamic instability

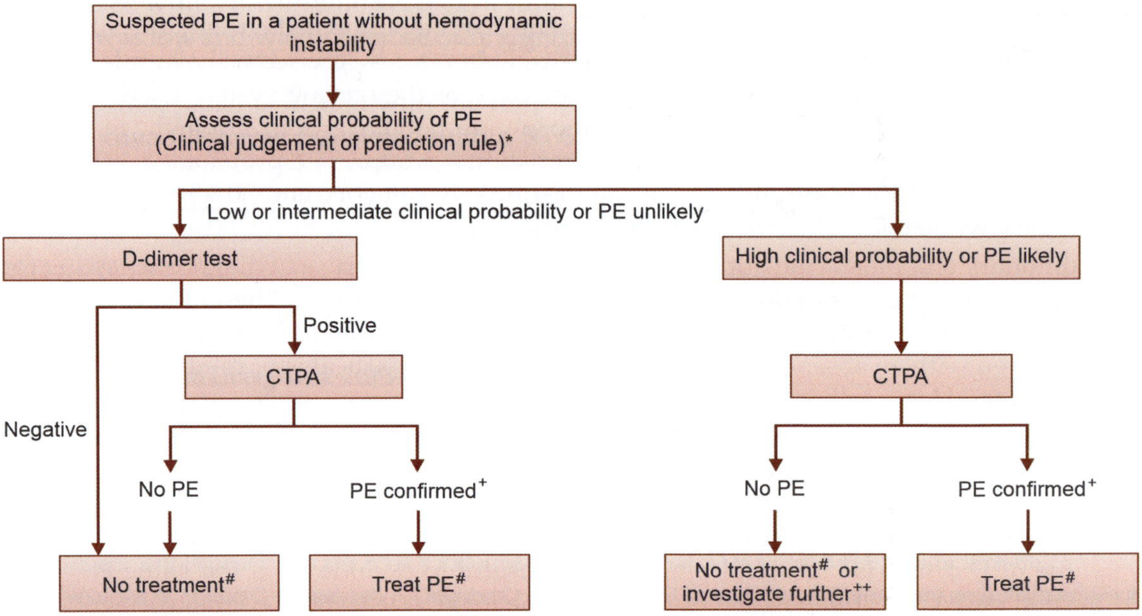

CTPA = Computed tomography pulmonary angiography/angiogram; PE = Pulmonary embolism.

*For clinical probability assessment, any of the two classification schemes can be used, i.e. a three-level scheme (clinical probability defined as low, intermediate, or high) or a two-level scheme (PE unlikely or PE likely). When using a moderately sensitive assay, use of D-dimer measurement should be limited to patients with low clinical probability or a PE-unlikely classification, while highly sensitive assays may also be used in patients with intermediate clinical probability of PE. Note that plasma D-dimer measurement is of limited value in hospitalized patients suspected of having PE.

#Treatment refers to anticoagulation treatment for PE.

+CTPA is considered diagnostic of PE if it demonstrates embolus at the segmental or more proximal level.

++In patients with high clinical probability and negative CTPA, further investigation using imaging may be considered before discontinuing PE-specific treatment.

g. *Compression ultrasonography*: PE usually originates from DVT in lower limb and rarely from DVT in upper limb. The use of compression ultrasonography has largely replaced venography as a modality to diagnose DVT with a sensitivity >90% and a specificity >95% for proximal symptomatic DVT.[10,11] In around 30–50% patients with PE, bedside compression sonography shows a DVT (10–12) and if there is presence of a proximal DVT, therapeutic anticoagulation can be initiated without further testing.[13]

Treatment

Treatment is primarily based on the risk category of the patient (Table 17.1). Reperfusion therapy along with anticoagulation is the modality of treatment in high risk category patients and intermediate high risk group with acute deterioration while therapeutic anticoagulation alone is the recommended approach for other categories.

a. *High risk patients*: Volume optimization using normal saline or lactated Ringer's in a volume of around 500 ml administered over 15–30 minutes, use of inotropes and vasopressors preferably Norepinephrine or Dopamine and mechanical circulatory support using VA ECMO/ECLS is the main approach for hemodynamic and respiratory support. In patients with right ventricular failure, systemic thrombolytic therapy results in earlier resolution of pulmonary obstruction compared with UFH alone. These improvements occur in parallel

Flowchart 17.2: Algorithm for diagnosis of PE in patients with hemodynamic instability

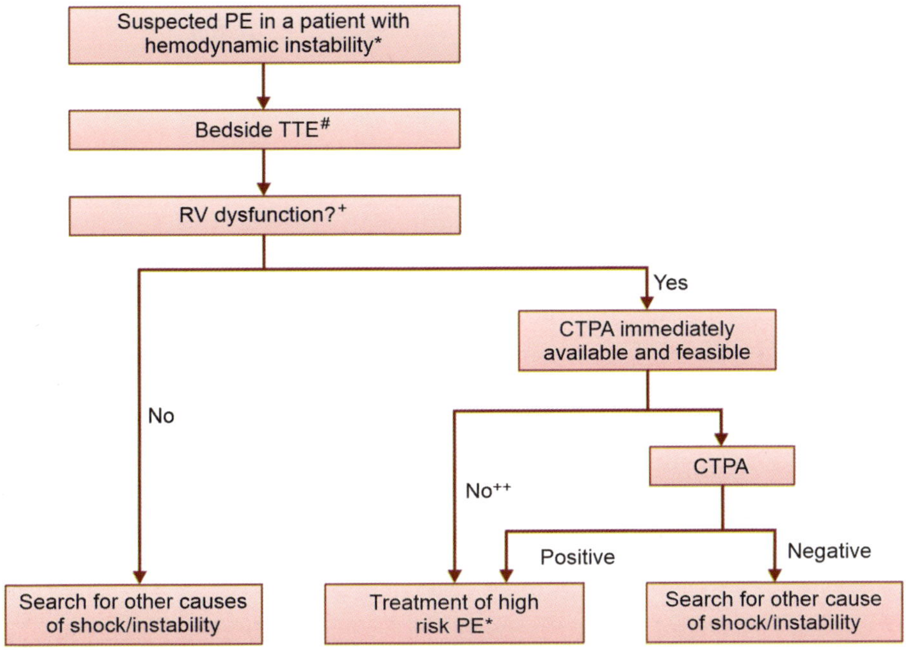

CTPA = Computed tomography pulmonary angiography; CUS = Compression ultrasonography; DVT = Deep vein thrombosis; PE = Pulmonary embolism; RV = Right ventricle; TOE = Transesophageal echocardiography; TTE = Transthoracic echocardiogram.

*one of the following clinical features: Cardiac arrest (need for cardiopulmonary resuscitation) OR obstructive shock [systolic BP <90 mmHg or vasopressors required to achieve a systolic BP of 90 mmHg or more, despite adequate intravascular volume status and features of end-organ hypoperfusion (altered mental status; cold, clammy skin; oliguria/anuria; increased serum lactate)] OR persistent hypotension [associate with end-organ hypoperfusion (altered mental status; cold, clammy skin; oliguria/anuria; increased serum lactate)]

#Ancillary bedside imaging tests may include TOE, which may detect emboli in the pulmonary artery and its main branches; and bilateral venous compression sonography, which may demonstrate DVT and thus VTE.

+The emergency scenario of suspected high-risk PE, which refers mainly to a RV/LV diameter ratio >1.0; the echocardiographic findings of RV dysfunction.

++Includes the clinical scenario in which the patient is critically ill and thus only bedside diagnostic tests can be performed. In such cases, echocardiographic findings of RV dysfunction confirm high-risk PE and emergency reperfusion therapy is recommended.

with resolution of RV dilatation.[14,15] The dosages and regimens for systemic thrombolytic therapy is predefined (Table 17.2). Initiation of treatment within 48 hours of symptom onset leads to greatest benefit, but thrombolytic therapy can still be helpful in patients who have had symptoms for the duration of 6 to 14 days.[16]

b. *Intermediate risk*: Anticoagulants should be started after suspecting PE in patients with intermediate risk and continued till confirmation of PE. If a patient with intermediate high risk deteriorates hemodynamically, then reperfusion therapy may be useful. Anticoagulants alone is sufficient for patients with intermediate low risk.
c. *Low risk*: Anticoagulants alone will suffice for patients with low risk with confirmed PE.
d. Choice of anticoagulants:
   i. *Parenteral anticoagulants*: In patients with high or intermediate clinical probability of PE, anticoagulation should be initiated while awaiting the results of the diagnostic tests. Either subcutaneous low molecular weight heparin (LMWH) or Fondaparinux or UFH

Table 17.1: Pulmonary embolism severity classification and risk of early (in-hospital or 0 day) mortality

Risk of early mortality		*Indicators of risk*			
		Hemodynamic instability	*Clinical parameters of PE severity and/or co-morbidity: PESI class III–IV or SPESI >= 1*	*TTE or CTPA showing RV dysfunction*	*Elevated levels of cardiac troponin*
High		+	(+)*	+	+
Intermediate	**High**	–	+#	+	+
	Low	–	+#	One or none positive	
Low		–	–	–	Assessment optional (if assessed negative)

(*)–Haemodynamically unstable patients, combined with CTPA confirmed PE and/or presence of RV dysfunction on TTE, is sufficient to label a patient in high-risk PE category. In these patients, calculation of the PESI, or measurement of troponins or other cardiac biomarkers is not necessary.

(#)–Signs of RV dysfunction on TTE (or CTPA) or elevated cardiac biomarker levels may be present, despite a calculated PESI of I–II or an sPESI of 0. These patients should be classified into the intermediate-risk category.

Table 17.2: Thrombolytic regimens along with their dosages

Molecule	*Regimen*
rtPA	• 100 mg over 2 h • Accelerated regimen: 0.6 mg/kg over 15 min (maximum dose 50 mg)*
Streptokinase	• 250000 IU as a loading dose over 30 min, followed by 100000 IU/h over 12–24 h • Accelerated regimen: 1.5 million IU over 2 h
Urokinase	• 4400 IU/kg as a loading dose over 10 min, followed by 4400 IU/kg/h over 12–24 h • Accelerated regimen: 3 million IU over 2 h

BP = blood pressure; IU = international units; rtPA = recombinant tissue-type plasminogen activator.

*This regimen is not approved officially, however, it is sometimes used in extremely unstable patients such as during cardiac arrest.

can be used as the initial regimen. LMWH and Fondaparinux are preferred over UFH as the former is associated with a lower risk of heparin-induced thrombocytopenia and major bleeding episodes.[17,18] A non-vitamin K antagonist oral anticoagulant (NOAC) can be used to attain equally rapid anticoagulation. Phase III clinical trials have shown non-inferiority of higher doses of apixaban (for 7 days) or rivaroxaban (for 3 weeks) when compared with conventional regimen.[19–21]

ii. *Non-vitamin K antagonist Oral anticoagulants*: These agents inhibit one of the activated coagulation factors in the coagulation cascade. Dabigatran directly inhibits thrombin. Agents like Rivaroxaban, Edoxaban and Apixaban inhibit factor Xa. The advantage of using NOACS are their predictable bioavailability, no requirement of routine laboratory monitoring and less drug interactions.

iii. *Vitamin K antagonists*: For decades, this has been the gold standard for oral anticoagulation. If VKAs are used for anticoagulation, then LMWH, UFH or Fondaparinux should be used concomitantly along with VKAs for 5 days or longer until the INR of 2–3 is attained for two consecutive days. The starting dose is 10 mg in otherwise healthy individuals aged <= 60 yrs and <= 5 mg in elderly patients. The daily dose is adjusted over the next 5 to 7 days which is guided by INR level with the aim to attain the level of 2.0–3.0.

iv. *Vena cava filters*: The aim of using these devices is to avoid clot from lower extremities to embolize to the pulmonary circulation. These devices are usually inserted and placed percutaneously. It can be considered in patients with VTE in whom anticoagulation is contraindicated, patients developing recurrent PE despite on adequate anticoagulation, and as a primary prophylaxis for patients who are at high risk of VTE.

EVIDENCE CONTOUR

a. *CT pulmonary angiography*: In the prospective investigation on pulmonary embolism diagnosis (PIOPED) II study, CTPA had the sensitivity of 83% and specificity of 96% for the diagnosis of PE.[5] RV dysfunction can be detected by visualizing enlargement of RV in the four-chamber view of the heart while performing CT angiography. Presence of increased RV end-diastolic diameter and RV/LV ratio indicates RV dysfunction. Presence of RV enlargement has prognostic significance, as observed in a prospective multicentre study involving over 450 patients.[22] It was observed that presence of RV enlargement which is defined as increased RV to LV ratio (0.9 or more) was independently associated with poor in hospital outcome. The outcome was unfavorable for both the overall population with PE [hazard ratio (HR) 3.5, 95% CI 1.67.7] and in patients without hemodynamic instability (HR 3.8, 95% CI 1.310.9).[22] Also, a meta-analysis of 49 studies involving over 13000 patients with PE showed that an increased RV/LV ratio (1.0 or more) as observed in CT was associated with a 2.5 times increased risk for all-cause mortality, and a five times increased risk of mortality associated with PE.[23]

b. *Reperfusion therapy*: In a meta-analysis of trials involving use of thrombolysis in patients with PE and cardiogenic shock, that also included the high-risk PE patients, thrombolysis was associated with significant reduction of both mortality and recurrence of PE. Use of thrombolysis was associated with 9.9% risk of severe bleeding and 1.7% risk of intracranial hemorrhage.[24] In the patients at intermediate risk for PE and who were normotensive, the role of thrombolytic therapy was investigated in the pulmonary embolism thrombolysis (PEITHO) trial. Intermediate risk was described as the patients with RV dysfunction and elevation of troponin levels.[25] Thrombolysis was associated with a significant reduction in hemodynamic instability, but was associated with elevated risk of both intracranial and extracranial hemorrhage.[25] In the PEITHO trial, in both the treatment groups, the 30-day mortality was low. However, subsequent meta-analysis of trials have suggested up to 50 to 60% reduction in overall and PE related mortality in patients at intermediate risk group.[24,26]

c. *Anticoagulants*: Studies have compared NOACs with the combination of LMWH with VKA. For both the treatment of acute incidence of VTE and for the extended treatment (beyond the initial 6 months), NOACs were found to be non-inferior to the combination of LMWH and VKA for the prevention of recurrence of VTE. However, NOACs were associated with reduced risk of major hemorrhagic complications.[27]

d. *Vena cava filters*: The prevention of recurrent pulmonary embolism by vena cava interruption (PREPIC) study evaluated the role of permanent vena cava filter in patients with PE. Use of vena cava filter was associated with a significantly reduced risk of recurrent PE but without any difference in the rates of VTE or mortality.[28] In the PREPIC-2 trial, patients with PE and DVT were randomized to be treated with either anticoagulation alone or with a retrievable vena cava filter. In both the groups, the rate of recurrence of VTE was low and was not statistically significant.[29] A systematic review and meta-analysis evaluating the efficacy and safety of vena cava filters that involved over 4000 patients from 11 studies, patients treated with the filter were compared with the controls.[30] The use of vena cava filter was associated with a 50% reduction in the incidence of PE, but with a 70% rise in the rates of DVT. However, PE associated mortality and all-cause mortality did not differ in those two groups.

REFERENCES

1. Shopp JD, Stewart LK, Emmett TW, Kline JA. Findings From 12-lead Electrocardiography That Predict Circulatory Shock From Pulmonary Embolism: Systematic Review and Meta-analysis. Acad Emerg Med Off J Soc Acad Emerg Med. 2015 Oct;22(10):1127–37.
2. Ceriani E, Combescure C, Le Gal G, Nendaz M, Perneger T, Bounameaux H, et al. Clinical prediction rules for pulmonary embolism: a systematic review and meta-analysis. J Thromb Haemost. 2010 May;8(5):957–70.
3. Freund Y, Cachanado M, Aubry A, Orsini C, Raynal P-A, Féral-Pierssens A-L, et al. Effect of the Pulmonary Embolism Rule-Out Criteria on Subsequent Thromboembolic Events Among Low-Risk Emergency Department Patients: The PROPER Randomized Clinical Trial. JAMA. 2018 Feb;319(6):559–66.
4. Penaloza A, Soulié C, Moumneh T, Delmez Q, Ghuysen A, El Kouri D, et al. Pulmonary embolism rule-out criteria (PERC) rule in European patients with low implicit clinical probability (PERCEPIC): a multicentre, prospective, observational study. Lancet Haematol. 2017 Dec;4(12):e615–21.
5. Stein PD, Fowler SE, Goodman LR, Gottschalk A, Hales CA, Hull RD, et al. Multidetector computed tomography for acute pulmonary embolism. N Engl J Med. 2006 Jun;354(22):2317–27.
6. Roy P-M, Colombet I, Durieux P, Chatellier G, Sors H, Meyer G. Systematic review and meta-analysis of strategies for the diagnosis of suspected pulmonary embolism. BMJ. 2005 Jul;331(7511):259.
7. Kurzyna M, Torbicki A, Pruszczyk P, Burakowska B, Fijałkowska A, Kober J, et al. Disturbed right ventricular ejection pattern as a new Doppler echocardiographic sign of acute pulmonary embolism. Am J Cardiol. 2002 Sep;90(5):507–11.
8. Pruszczyk P, Goliszek S, Lichodziejewska B, Kostrubiec M, Ciurzyński M, Kurnicka K, et al. Prognostic value of echocardiography in normotensive patients with acute pulmonary embolism. JACC Cardiovasc Imaging. 2014 Jun;7(6):553–60.
9. Dresden S, Mitchell P, Rahimi L, Leo M, Rubin-Smith J, Bibi S, et al. Right ventricular dilatation on bedside echocardiography performed by emergency physicians aids in the diagnosis of pulmonary embolism. Ann Emerg Med. 2014 Jan;63(1):16–24.
10. Perrier A, Bounameaux H. Ultrasonography of leg veins in patients suspected of having pulmonary embolism. Vol. 128, Annals of internal medicine. United States; 1998. p. 243; author reply 244–5.
11. Kearon C, Ginsberg JS, Hirsh J. The role of venous ultrasonography in the diagnosis of suspected deep venous thrombosis and pulmonary embolism. Ann Intern Med. 1998 Dec;129(12):1044–9.
12. Righini M, Le Gal G, Aujesky D, Roy P-M, Sanchez O, Verschuren F, et al. Diagnosis of pulmonary embolism by multidetector CT alone or combined with venous ultrasonography of the leg: a randomised non-inferiority trial. Lancet (London, England). 2008 Apr;371(9621):1343–52.
13. Le Gal G, Righini M, Sanchez O, Roy P-M, Baba-Ahmed M, Perrier A, et al. A positive compression ultrasonography of the lower limb veins is highly predictive of pulmonary embolism on computed tomography in suspected patients. Thromb Haemost. 2006 Jun;95(6):963–6.
14. Timp JF, Braekkan SK, Versteeg HH, Cannegieter SC. Epidemiology of cancer-associated venous thrombosis. Blood. 2013 Sep;122(10):1712–23.
15. White RH. The epidemiology of venous thromboembolism. Circulation. 2003 Jun;107(23 Suppl 1):I4–8.
16. Raskob GE, Angchaisuksiri P, Blanco AN, Buller H, Gallus A, Hunt BJ, et al. Thrombosis: a major contributor to global disease burden. Arterioscler Thromb Vasc Biol. 2014 Nov;34(11):2363–71.

17. Erkens PM, Prins MH. Fixed dose subcutaneous low molecular weight heparins versus adjusted dose unfractionated heparin for venous thromboembolism. Cochrane database Syst Rev. 2010 Sep;(9):CD001100.
18. Cossette B, Pelletier M-E, Carrier N, Turgeon M, Leclair C, Charron P, et al. Evaluation of bleeding risk in patients exposed to therapeutic unfractionated or low-molecular-weight heparin: a cohort study in the context of a quality improvement initiative. Ann Pharmacother. 2010 Jun;44(6):994–1002.
19. Steffel J, Verhamme P, Potpara TS, Albaladejo P, Antz M, Desteghe L, et al. The 2018 European Heart Rhythm Association Practical Guide on the use of non-vitamin K antagonist oral anticoagulants in patients with atrial fibrillation. Eur Heart J. 2018 Apr;39(16):1330–93.
20. Agnelli G, Buller HR, Cohen A, Curto M, Gallus AS, Johnson M, et al. Oral apixaban for the treatment of acute venous thromboembolism. N Engl J Med. 2013 Aug;369(9):799–808.
21. Büller HR, Prins MH, Lensin AWA, Decousus H, Jacobson BF, Minar E, et al. Oral rivaroxaban for the treatment of symptomatic pulmonary embolism. N Engl J Med. 2012 Apr;366(14):1287–97.
22. Becattini C, Agnelli G, Vedovati MC, Pruszczyk P, Casazza F, Grifoni S, et al. Multidetector computed tomography for acute pulmonary embolism: diagnosis and risk stratification in a single test. Eur Heart J. 2011 Jul;32(13):1657–63.
23. Meinel FG, Nance JWJ, Schoepf UJ, Hoffmann VS, Thierfelder KM, Costello P, et al. Predictive Value of Computed Tomography in Acute Pulmonary Embolism: Systematic Review and Meta-analysis. Am J Med. 2015 Jul;128(7):747-59.e2.
24. Marti C, John G, Konstantinides S, Combescure C, Sanchez O, Lankeit M, et al. Systemic thrombolytic therapy for acute pulmonary embolism: a systematic review and meta-analysis. Eur Heart J. 2015 Mar;36(10):605–14.
25. Meyer G, Vicaut E, Danays T, Agnelli G, Becattini C, Beyer-Westendorf J, et al. Fibrinolysis for patients with intermediate-risk pulmonary embolism. N Engl J Med. 2014 Apr;370(15):1402–11.
26. Chatterjee S, Chakraborty A, Weinberg I, Kadakia M, Wilensky RL, Sardar P, et al. Thrombolysis for pulmonary embolism and risk of all-cause mortality, major bleeding, and intracranial hemorrhage: a meta-analysis. JAMA. 2014 Jun;311(23):2414–21.
27. van Es N, Coppens M, Schulman S, Middeldorp S, Büller HR. Direct oral anticoagulants compared with vitamin K antagonists for acute venous thromboembolism: evidence from phase 3 trials. Blood. 2014 Sep;124(12):1968–75.
28. Decousus H, Leizorovicz A, Parent F, Page Y, Tardy B, Girard P, et al. A clinical trial of vena caval filters in the prevention of pulmonary embolism in patients with proximal deep-vein thrombosis. Prévention du Risque d'Embolie Pulmonaire par Interruption Cave Study Group. N Engl J Med. 1998 Feb;338(7):409–15.
29. Mismetti P, Laporte S, Pellerin O, Ennezat P-V, Couturaud F, Elias A, et al. Effect of a retrievable inferior vena cava filter plus anticoagulation vs anticoagulation alone on risk of recurrent pulmonary embolism: a randomized clinical trial. JAMA. 2015 Apr;313(16):1627–35.
30. Bikdeli B, Chatterjee S, Desai NR, Kirtane AJ, Desai MM, Bracken MB, et al. Inferior Vena Cava Filters to Prevent Pulmonary Embolism: Systematic Review and Meta-Analysis. J Am Coll Cardiol. 2017 Sep;70(13):1587–97.

CHAPTER

18

Biomarker Guided Antibiotic Therapy

Shashi Bhaskara Krishnamurthy, Divya Shetty

CASE DESCRIPTION

A 46-year-old male was admitted to the ICU with community acquired pneumonia. He has a background history of recently diagnosed lung cancer. He has been a smoker in the past and consumes alcohol once a week. He had a infusor port for chemotherapy and had completed a cycle of chemotherapy 5 days prior to admission. At presentation in the emergency department he was mildly confused, had a RR 25/min, BP 100/60 mmHg, SpO_2 87% on room air that improved to 92% with O_2 via face mask @ 4L/min. He was initiated on IV Ceftriaxone 500 mg once daily, IV Azithromycin 500 mg IV once daily as antibiotics for his illness. He was initially admitted on the wards. However, on day 4 of his illness, he became tachypnoeic and had to be transferred to the ICU for initiation of NIV. He was soon invasively ventilated for features suggesting ARDS and required inotropes for shock. Cultures were sent for new onset fevers. Investigations revealed that his total count had increased to 23000/cumm with neutrophil left shift, CRP 56 mg/dL, procalcitonin 12 ng/mL. CXR showed a new patch on the left side. With a diagnosis of a new hospital acquired pneumonia antibiotics were escalated to Meropenem and Vancomycin. After 4 days of supportive care, he improved clinically with reducing FiO_2, inotropes and no fevers. Repeat CRP on day 9 was 22 mg/dL and Procalcitonin had reduced to 4 ng/L. Endotracheal secretion culture was reported as *E. coli* sensitive to Piperacillin and Tazobactum and hence antibiotics were de-escalated.

What is the best approach that can be used to choose antibiotics with a suspected community acquired pneumonia in this patient when he presents to the hospital?

- Risk stratification—PSI scoring, CURB 65 score, etc.
- Initiating antibiotics using biomarker guided approach as a tool
- Choosing broad spectrum antibiotics—local guidelines.

The choice of antibiotics for infection and sepsis is guided by broad spectrum empirical treatment guidelines and PK/PD parameters. Following empirical antibiotics, the course of action taken by physicians includes identification of sources using tools such as an adequate history, focussed examination and investigations. Choosing the antibiotic is based on the local guidelines after risk stratification such as PSI score or CURB 65 score for illnesses such as pneumonia. The next step in management would be source control. This is especially true if there is a localised source such as a collection or abscess that is amenable to surgical debridement or evacuation. The empirical antibiotics can then be narrowed down to targeted antibiotics on the availability of cultures.

Most of the infections respond to the empirical course or to the antibiotics depending on culture and sensitivity. However, there are variations in the treatment response such as treatment failure due to either pathogen specific reasons such as antibiotic resistance or patient specific reasons such as the drug-induced organ damage or other adverse events.[1]

Recommendation from sepsis and other guidelines is to use antibiotics early, of appropriate dose and for the shortest duration possible, however, a lot of these are left to the discretion of the treating physician.[4]

There are two main strategies to individualise antibiotic drug treatment that are effective on the targets such as 'therapeutic drug monitoring', 'biomarker-based strategy'.[1] Therapeutic drug monitoring helps to individualise drug treatment based on predefined targets with respect to efficacy and prevention of toxicity. Many a times, infections like respiratory tract infections so not yield samples for cultures or often remain sterile. Prior exposure to antibiotics may also alter the culture results. Hence, we may be left with no laboratory tool to guide therapy and stewardship. Biomarkers help to further rationalise antibiotic treatment with respect to efficacy, toxicity and reduce the incidence of antibiotic resistance.

What is a biomarker and how should biomarkers be used in clinical practice for management of infection?

One of the first definitions of biomarker came from the 1998 National Institute of Health Biomarkers Definitions Working Group defined biomarkers as "a characteristic that is objectively measured and evaluated as an indicator of normal biological processes, pathogenic processes or pharmacological responses to a therapeutic intervention".[2] This has been followed by more iterations of the definition and an accepted definition of biomarkers for guiding antibiotic therapy is that they are measurable proteins or other chemicals produced from cells and tissues as a response triggered by the immune system when a patient is exposed to bacteria. Apart from recognition of a disease, they would also help physicians to predict risk, identify disease progression, biologically effective dose determination, clinical effects of treatments, interventions, toxicity either from the bacteria or the intervention.[2,3] The best approach to its use and relationships to clinical endpoints is still being developed and perfected. In practice, normalising the laboratory value of the biomarker must not be the goal of patient management, but improving the clinical endpoint such as morbidity and mortality must be given a highest importance.

What biomarkers can be used while deciding the host response to an infection?

The biomarkers available for clinical decision making include procalcitonin, CRP (C reactive protein), IL-6 (Interleukin 6), Presepsin, (soluble) triggering receptor expressed on myeloid cells 1 (sTREM-1), tumour necrosis factor-α (TNF-α). Lipopolysaccharide (LPS).

Procalcitonin: Is the precursor of calcitonin produced by the parafollicular cells of thyroid cells. In response to exposure to bacteria, procalcitonin is induced throughout the body where it is thought to have immune modulatory effects. It is inhibited by interferon-γ and hence there is minimal elevation in viral illnesses.

This is the only biomarker that has been extensively studied from an antibiotic stewardship point of view and has been very promising to help clinicians guide antibiotic therapy. Studies in patients with respiratory tract infections and sepsis[1,5] has reliably resulted in its use for guiding antibiotic duration. Studies show that procalcitonin guided therapy significantly reduces in hospital mortality,[5] but not reduction in hospital length of stay or 28-day mortality, recurrence of infection or readmission.[1,5]

C Reactive Protein (CRP): It is an acute phase protein released by the hepatocytes in response to an infection. It activates the complement pathway and plays a role in the innate immune response.

CRP secretion is initiated within 4–6 hours of infection and doubles every 8 hours. The levels are proportional to the inflammatory insult.[9] The levels are reduced when there is a clinical response to an antibiotic,[1] however, admission CRP level does not predict outcomes in sepsis or respiratory tract infections.

Interleukin-6: It is a cytokine released by immune cells as a response to infection. It is both a pro-inflammatory and anti-inflammatory cytokine and quantifies disease severity.

Presepsin: It is a product of CD14 membrane and it is involved in innate immune response and bacterial phagocytosis. It is released with host exposure to both bacterial and fungal infections. Presepsin levels correlate with severity of sepsis as well as predict mortality and survival.

Soluble Triggering Receptors Expressed in Myeloid cells (sTREM-1): These are released by the host cells in response to bacterial and fungal exposure. In suspected infection, it is more clinically significant to measure sTREM from sites of infection such as CSF, BAL, pleural fluid than plasma.[6]

Pro-Adrenomedullin (proADM): It is a biomarker released by the endothelial cells in response to infection. It is a biomarker that can be used to identify patients with community acquired pneumonia who need closer monitoring and ICU admission.[12]

Soluble urokinase-type plasminogen activator receptor (suPAR) OR CD87: It is released by endothelium or leukocytes in response to immune or inflammation as well as during tumour growth and metastasis. Its significance appears to be in HIV patients with the presence of non-pulmonary mycobacterium tuberculosis, however, its use in clinical practice is limited.

There are several other biomarkers involved with inflammation and organ damage in general.

There are changes in the levels of proteins, platelets and other components of the blood as an acute phase reaction of the body to exposure to stress.[2,3]

How do we decide what biomarker should be used in which context?

Biomarkers can be used to individualise treatment depending upon the host response to the organism or intervention by the use of antibiotics.

There are detectable levels of biomarkers such as presepsin, sTREM within 2 hours; procalcitonin within 3–4 hours; and CRP by 4–6 hours after exposure to the pathogen.[1,6,9] CRP and procalcitonin are the two most widely studied and used biomarkers for guiding antibiotics.[9] Biomarkers can also be used for quantifying the antibiotic response in sepsis.

CRP when used in primary care is one of the best biomarkers for infection and extent of inflammation.[9] Despite having several inter-patient variability in its response, serial levels of procalcitonin can be used in clinical practice to understand severity of sepsis and the host response to the antibiotic.

Procalcitonin along with lipopolysaccharide has a more quantitative relationship with gram negative organisms than gram positive organisms.[11] Procalcitonin aids initiation and or discontinuation of antibiotics in children and adults and can be used from primary care, emergency departments, wards and ICU.[9] A decline in the levels indicates that the treatment is effective and the rate of decrease indicates treatment specificity.

Procalcitonin seems to be the biomarker most studied and shown to be most beneficial for guiding antibiotic therapy for secondary bacterial infection during COVID-19 infection.[6] Procalcitonin levels are less affected by either the hyperinflammation due to COVID or by the immunomodulatory treatment unlike CRP that is affected by both. Since most of the infections with COVID-19 occur after admission, it would be useful to start antibiotics when the procalcitonin levels rise to > 1 ng/mL and withhold antibiotics when levels drop to <25 ng/mL. The total number of patients studied with respect to biomarker guided antibiotics in COVID is small compared to the number of patients affected with COVID worldwide, nevertheless, this is shown to reduce 28-day mortality, reduce intubation and ICU admission rates.[6]

Further, biomarkers can guide the efficacy and toxicity during the ongoing phase and ending of treatment with the antibiotic.[1] Biomarkers with prolonged half life would be of less clinical value. Pathogens can have effect on hepatic or renal clearance and the clearance of some biomarkers such as CRP or IL-6 also depends on this systemic clearance and hence can be used to predict inflammation of liver or the kidney.

Antibiotics exposure causes toxicity, however when guided by biomarkers, there would be safer treatments and reduction of morbidity and mortality. To date, use of therapeutic drug monitoring is the only available static measure to predict individuals exposure to toxicities and organ dysfunction. Further correlation with indicators such as creatinine or liver enzymes can be used to monitor organ function during exposure to antibiotics. The baseline concentration of platelets can predict haematological toxicity after exposure to Linezolid.[13] In clinical practice, other biomarkers are of limited availability. Some examples include use of a panel such as cystatin-c, kidney injury molecule-1 and NGAL can be used for treatment monitoring and prevention of nephrotoxicity.[14] Procalcitonin guided antibiotic use can also be used to reduce the incidence of diarrhoea and acute kidney injury (AKI).[6]

Although liver enzymes are markers of hepatotoxicity, they do not correlate to dynamic changes. Glutamate dehydrogenase with a half life of 11–18 hours and microRNA based biomarkers play an important role as a biomarker in identifying antibiotic induced liver damage.[1]

Biomarkers have a role in the development of drugs and this might occur while treating infections in critically ill patients.[1] During these circumstances, one must be careful with the reliance or overreliance on the biomarkers as the surrogate end point and continue managing patients based on expected course of illness, pathophysiological processes and clinical endpoints.

How do biomarkers help in decision making about the duration of therapy with antibiotics?

Biomarker guided antibiotic treatment algorithms help in antibiotic initiation and cessation, thus reducing the incidence of complications associated with its use.[6] However, there is no evidence to back up that such algorithms reduce readmission rates due to infection.

Such decisions are backed up by plenty of evidence specifically with reference to use of procalcitonin to guide treatment. It can be used for deciding the timing of initiation (when levels are >0.25 ng/mL, repeat levels on day[3,5,7] and discontinuation of an antibiotic when levels fall below 0.5 ng/ml or drop by 80–90%).[10] Hence, it can be included in the decision algorithms for community acquired lower respiratory tract infections.[1,5,6] Studies have used algorithms when serial measurements of procalcitonin at baseline, day[3,5,7] led to earlier discontinuation of antibiotics[7,8,10] as well as long term infectious complications such as new infection with multidrug resistant organisms, C diff and mortality.[6]

Other biomarkers such as CRP and presepsin have also been found to reduce the duration of antibiotics and not the mortality. A reduction of CRP by 50% or <35 mg/dL can be used to stop antibiotics therapy.[6] Presepsin has an advantage that it rises within 2 hours of an infection and a reduction to <350 pg/mL or more than 80% from baseline can be used to stop the antibiotic.[6] The access to presepsis as a point of care analysis and minimal turnaround time for clinical applicability is limited.

It is important to note that by reducing the duration of antibiotics using biomarker guided antibiotic algorithms there is no increased mortality, hence, it would be safe to use this strategy and prevent antibiotic related toxicity and complications from prolonged use of antibiotics.

Also, SAPS study showed a reduction in cost of treatment when procalcitonin was used for guiding antibiotics.[8] This is especially relevant in low and middle income countries when the cost implications play an important role in patient management.

What are the controversial aspects of management using biomarkers to guide antibiotic therapy?

While measuring biomarkers, there is a concern with regard to inter-individual variability due to various factors such as amount of exposure, laboratory errors, individual differences in expression of the effects of the pathogen or metabolism of the biomarkers.[3]

The use of procalcitonin does not show effectiveness in secondary outcomes such as hospital length of stay, 28-day mortality and recurrence of infection or rehospitalisation.[5]

However, adherence to biomarker based treatment protocols in a practical setting is challenging due to difficulty in interpretation.[5] Further, there is limited evidence with respect to biomarker guided antibiotics in the immunosuppressed patients[4] where the need for such information is paramount.

Procalcitonin levels are increased among patients with non-infectious conditions such as trauma, burns, cancers, immunomodulator therapy and patients with CKD.[10]

In conclusion, using biomarkers as an essential tool for antibiotic stewardship helps in objectively distinguishing patients who will benefit from starting antibiotics with the suspicion of infection. It will also lead to limited use of antibiotics thus reducing complications of morbidity, mortality, resistance as well as cost reduction.

REFERENCES

1. Aulin LBS, de Lange DW, Saleh MAA, van der Graaf PH, Völler S, van Hasselt JGC. Biomarker-Guided Individualization of Antibiotic Therapy. Clin Pharmacol Ther. 2021 Aug;110(2):346-360. doi: 10.1002/cpt.2194. Epub 2021 Mar 2. PMID: 33559152; PMCID: PMC8359228.
2. Biomarkers Definition Working Group. Biomarkers and surrogate endpoints: preferred definitions and conceptual framework. Clin Pharmacol Therapeutics. 2001; 69:89–95.
3. Mayeux R. Biomarkers: potential uses and limitations. NeuroRx. 2004 Apr;1(2):182-8. doi: 10.1602/neurorx.1.2.182. PMID: 15717018; PMCID: PMC534923.
4. Dupuy AM, Philippart F, Péan Y, Lasocki S, Charles PE, Chalumeau M, Claessens YE, Quenot JP, Guen CG, Ruiz S, Luyt CE, Roche N, Stahl JP, Bedos JP, Pugin J, Gauzit R, Misset B, Brun-Buisson C; Maurice Rapin Institute Biomarkers Group. Role of biomarkers in the management of antibiotic therapy: an expert panel review: I - currently available biomarkers for clinical use in acute infections. Ann Intensive Care. 2013 Jul 9;3(1):22. doi: 10.1186/2110-5820-3-22. PMID: 23837559; PMCID: PMC3708786.
5. Elnajdy D, El-Dahiyat F. Antibiotics duration guided by biomarkers in hospitalised adult patients; a systematic review and meta-analysis. Infect Dis (Lond). 2022 Jun;54(6):387-402. doi: 10.1080/23744235.2022.2037701. Epub 2022 Feb 17. PMID: 35175169.

6. Kyriazopoulou, E.; Giamarellos-Bourboulis, E.J. Antimicrobial Stewardship Using Biomarkers: Accumulating Evidence for the Critically Ill. Antibiotics 2022, 11, 367. https://doi.org/10.3390/antibiotics11030367
7. Bouadma L, Luyt CE, Tubach F, Cracco C, Alvarez A, Schwebel C, Schortgen F, Lasocki S, Veber B, Dehoux M, Bernard M, Pasquet B, Régnier B, Brun-Buisson C, Chastre J, Wolff M; PRORATA trial group. Use of procalcitonin to reduce patients' exposure to antibiotics in intensive care units (PRORATA trial): a multicentre randomised controlled trial. Lancet. 2010 Feb 6;375(9713):463–74. doi: 10.1016/S0140-6736(09)61879-1. Epub 2010 Jan 25. PMID: 20097417.
8. Assink-de Jong E, de Lange DW, van Oers JA, Nijsten MW, Twisk JW, Beishuizen A. Stop Antibiotics on guidance of Procalcitonin Study (SAPS): a randomised prospective multicenter investigator-initiated trial to analyse whether daily measurements of procalcitonin versus a standard-of-care approach can safely shorten antibiotic duration in intensive care unit patients--calculated sample size: 1816 patients. BMC Infect Dis. 2013 Apr 16;13:178. doi: 10.1186/1471-2334-13-178. PMID: 23590389; PMCID: PMC3637799.
9. Nora D, Salluh J, Martin-Loeches I, Póvoa P. Biomarker-guided antibiotic therapy—strengths and limitations. Ann Transl Med 2017;5(10):208. doi: 10.21037/atm.2017.04.04
10. Cleland DA, Eranki AP. Procalcitonin. [Updated 2022 Aug 8]. In: StatPearls [Internet]. Treasure Island (FL): StatPearls Publishing; 2022 Jan-. Available from: https://www.ncbi.nlm.nih.gov/books/NBK539794/
11. Oussalah A, Ferrand J, Filhine-Tresarrieu P, Aissa N, Aimone-Gastin I, Namour F, Garcia M, Lozniewski A, Guéant JL. Diagnostic Accuracy of Procalcitonin for Predicting Blood Culture Results in Patients With Suspected Bloodstream Infection: An Observational Study of 35,343 Consecutive Patients (A STROBE-Compliant Article). Medicine (Baltimore). 2015 Nov;94(44):e1774. doi: 10.1097/MD.0000000000001774. PMID: 26554775; PMCID: PMC4915876.
12. Bello S, Lasierra AB, Mincholé E, Fandos S, Ruiz MA, Vera E, de Pablo F, Ferrer M, Menendez R, Torres A. Prognostic power of proadrenomedullin in community-acquired pneumonia is independent of aetiology. Eur Respir J. 2012 May;39(5):1144-55. doi: 10.1183/09031936.00080411. Epub 2011 Nov 10. PMID: 22075489.
13. LiverTox: Clinical and Research Information on Drug-Induced Liver Injury [Internet]. Bethesda (MD): National Institute of Diabetes and Digestive and Kidney Diseases; 2012-. Linezolid. [Updated 2019 Jun 6]. Available from: https://www.ncbi.nlm.nih.gov/books/NBK548245/
14. van Duijl TT, Ruhaak LR, de Fijter JW, Cobbaert CM. Kidney Injury Biomarkers in an Academic Hospital Setting: Where Are We Now? Clin Biochem Rev. 2019 May;40(2):79–97. doi: 10.33176/AACB-18-00017. PMID: 31205376; PMCID: PMC6544249.

CHAPTER

19

Preventing and Managing Errors and Adverse Events in ICU

Quirino Piacevoli

This project was finalized to prevent and managing all the near misses and the clinical incidents in major hospitals in Italy.

Key Facts

- The occurrence of adverse events due to unsafe care is likely one of the 10 leading causes of death and disability in the world.
- In high-income countries, it is estimated that one in every 10 patients is harmed while receiving hospital care. The harm can be caused by a range of adverse events, with nearly 50% of them being preventable.
- Each year, 134 million adverse events occur in hospitals in low- and middle-income countries (LMICs), due to unsafe care, resulting in 2.6 million deaths.
- Another study has estimated that around two-thirds of all adverse events resulting from unsafe care, and the years lost to disability and death (known as disability adjusted life years, or DALYs) occur in LMICs.
- Globally, as many as 4 in 10 patients are harmed in primary and outpatient health care. Up to 80% of harm is preventable. The most detrimental errors are related to diagnosis, prescription, and the use of medicines.
- In OECD countries, 15% of total hospital activity and expenditure is a direct result of adverse events.
- Investments in reducing patient harm can lead to significant financial savings, and more importantly better patient outcomes. An example of prevention is engaging patients, if done well, it can reduce the burden of harm by up to 15%.
- Patient Safety is a health care discipline that emerged with the evolving complexity in health care systems and the resulting rise of patient harm in health care facilities. It aims to prevent and reduce risks, errors and harm that occur to patients during provision of health care. A cornerstone of the discipline is continuous improvement based on learning from errors and adverse events.
- Patient safety is fundamental to deliver quality essential health services. Indeed, there is a clear consensus that quality health services across the world should be effective, safe and people centred. In addition, to realize the benefits of quality health care, health services must be timely, equitable, integrated, and efficient.
- To ensure successful implementation of patient safety strategies clear policies, leadership capacity, data to drive safety improvements, skilled health care professionals and effective involvement of patients in their care, are all needed.

- A mature health system considers the increasing complexity in health care settings that make humans more prone to mistakes. For example, a patient in hospital might receive a wrong medication because of a mix-up that occurs due to similar packaging. In this case, the prescription passes through different levels of care starting with the doctor in the ward, then to the pharmacy for dispensing and finally to the nurse who administers the wrong medication to the patient. Had there been safeguarding processes in place at the different levels, this error could have been quickly identified and corrected. In this situation, a lack of standard procedures for storage of medications that look alike, poor communication between the different providers, lack of verification before medication administration and lack of involvement of patients in their own care might all be underlying factors that led to the occurrence of errors. Traditionally, the individual provider who actively made the mistake (active error) would take the blame for such an incident occurring and might also be punished as a result. Unfortunately, this does not consider the factors in the system previously described that led to the occurrence of error (latent errors). It is when multiple latent errors align that an active error reaches the patient.
- To err is human and expecting flawless performance from human beings working in complex, high-stress environments is unrealistic. Assuming that individual perfection is possible will not improve safety. Humans are guarded from making mistakes when placed in an error-proof environment where the systems, tasks and processes they work in are well designed. Therefore, focusing on the system that allows harm to occur is the beginning of improvement, and this can only occur in an open and transparent environment where a safety culture prevails. This is a culture where a high level of importance is placed on safety beliefs, values and attitudes and shared by most people within the workplace.

Every year, millions of patients suffer injuries or die because of unsafe and poor-quality health care. Many medical practices and risks associated with health care are emerging as major challenges for patient safety and contribute significantly to the burden of harm due to unsafe care. Below are some of the patient safety situations causing most concern.

Medication errors are a leading cause of injury and avoidable harm in health care systems: globally, the cost associated with medication errors has been estimated at US$ 42 billion annually.

Health care-associated infections occur in 7 and 10 out of every 100 hospitalized patients in high-income countries and low- and middle-income countries respectively.

Unsafe surgical care procedures cause complications in up to 25% of patients. Almost 7 million surgical patients suffer significant complications annually, 1 million of whom die during or immediately following surgery.

Unsafe injections practices in health care settings can transmit infections, including HIV and hepatitis B and C, and pose direct danger to patients and health care workers; they account for a burden of harm estimated at 9.2 million years of life lost to disability and death worldwide (known as Disability Adjusted Life Years (DALYs).

Diagnostic errors occur in about 5% of adults in outpatient care settings, more than half of which have the potential to cause severe harm. Most people will suffer a diagnostic error in their lifetime.

Unsafe transfusion practices expose patients to the risk of adverse transfusion reactions and the transmission of infections. Data on adverse transfusion reactions from a group of

21 countries show an average incidence of 8.7 serious reactions per 100 000 distributed blood components.

Radiation errors involve overexposure to radiation and cases of wrong-patient and wrong-site identification. A review of 30 years of published data on safety in radiotherapy estimates that the overall incidence of errors is around 15 per 10 000 treatment courses.

Sepsis is frequently not diagnosed early enough to save a patient's life. Because these infections are often resistant to antibiotics, they can rapidly lead to deteriorating clinical conditions, affecting an estimated 31 million people worldwide and causing over 5 million deaths per year.

Venous thromboembolism (blood clots) is one of the most common and preventable causes of patient harm, contributing to one-third of the complications attributed to hospitalization. Annually, there are an estimated 3.9 million cases in high-income countries and 6 million cases in low- and middle-income countries.

Patient Safety: A Fundamental Component for Universal Health Coverage

Resolution (WHA 72.6) on Patient Safety

Recognizing that Patient Safety is a global health priority, the World Health Assembly (WHA) adopted a resolution on Patient Safety which endorsed the establishment of World Patient Safety Day to be observed annually by Member States on 17 September.

1. Patient Safety as a global health priority
    - https://mailchi.mp/who.int/wha-72-achievements-commitment-accountability
    - https://www.who.int/patientsafety/policies/global-health-priority/en/
    - (WHA 72.6)

The purpose of World Patient Safety Day is to promote patient safety by increasing public awareness and engagement, enhancing global understanding, and working towards global solidarity and action.

Purposes of Reporting

An effective reporting system is the cornerstone of safe practice, and within a hospital or other health care organization, a measure of progress towards achieving a safety culture.

Why should individuals or health care organization report adverse events and errors?

If the event is reported and the findings from the investigation are entered into a database, the event can be aggregated with similar incidents to elucidate common underlying causes.

A variety of solutions could emerge, ranging from medical and nursing practice standards.

The Core concepts

Fundamental role of patient safety reporting systems is to announce patient safety by learning from failures of the health care system.

Reporting must be safe. Individuals who report incidences must not be punished or suffer other ill-effects from reporting.

Reporting is only of value if it leads to a constructive response.

Meaningful analysis, learning and dissemination of lessons learned require expertise and other human and financial resources.

Key Messages

The primary purpose of patient safety reporting system is to learn from the experience.

A reporting system must produce a visible, useful response to justify resources expended and to stimulate reporting.

The most important function of reporting system is to use the results of data analysis and investigation to formulate and disseminate recommendations for system change.

Components of Reporting System

A current reporting system span a spectrum of objectives incorporating both learning and accountability consideration.

The primary objectives of reporting system will determine the design, for example, whether reporting is voluntary and confidential.

Reporting systems need to be clear on who reports, the scope of what is reported and how reports are made.

Reposting of incidence is a little value unless the data collected are analyzed and recommendations are disseminated.

Experts are essential to analyse reported incidence.

Classification and simple analytic schemes start the process of categorizing the data and developing solutions that can be generalized.

What is Reported?

Adverse events: Is an injury related to medical management, in contrast to a complication of disease.

Errors: Has been defined as "the failure of a planned action to complete as intended or the use of a wrong plan to achieve an aim.

Near miss or close call is a serious error or mishap that has the potential to cause an adverse event but fails to do so by chance or because it was intercepted.

Hazards and unsafe condition are another way to achieve prevention without the need to learn from an injury.

SAFETY ASSESSMENT CODE MATRIX

Probability	*Severity*			
	Catastrophic	*Major*	*Moderate*	*Minor*
Frequent	16	12	8	4
Occasional	12	9	6	3
Uncommon	8	6	4	2
Remote	4	3	2	1

So, we suggested starting with a national/regional on-going project of total quality improvement in several Indian hospitals as soon as possible.

Risk management involving both patients and health care professionals is an important aspect of a total quality concept to:

- increase the standard of care
- improve efficiency in organization

- obtain better resource allocation
- reduce legal exposure

OBJECTIVES OF THE PROJECT

- To identify major risk factors in Italian hospitals
- To measure their frequency, we collected more than 70,000 events
- To identify causes and facilitating conditions
- To propose realistic solutions capable of reducing risks.

CHAPTER

20

Life-Threatening Metabolic and Electrolyte Disturbances

Kathryn Essak, Nitin Arora, Ahsina Jahan Lopa

ABSTRACT

Critically ill patients are frequently prone to electrolyte and metabolic disturbance. There are multiple etiologies for the same and the management protocol also varies. This chapter deals with two common metabolic and electrolyte disturbance frequently faced by intensivists and the proper way of diagnosis and management of such problems.

- ***Keywords:*** *DKA, Hyperkalemia, Rhabdomyolysis*

CASE

A 30-year-old male presented to the emergency department with type 1 respiratory failure and septic shock after a 5-day history of feeling generally unwell with fevers, productive cough, reduced oral intake and diarrhoea.

He was intubated and ventilated in resus and underwent thoracic CT imaging. This showed bilateral patchy infiltrates. He was found to have a positive covid PCR and raised inflammatory markers with marked neutrophilia.

Subsequently, the patient was treated as atypical pneumonia with a combination of piperacillin/tazobactam and levofloxacin. Aside from omeprazole administered for gastric protection, no other medications are being given.

He was proned shortly after admission to ITU, reducing his FIO_2 from 1.0 to 0.7 to maintain saturations of 94% with lung protective airway pressures. His vasopressor requirement was improving and FIO_2 improved to 0.4 after 72 hours and three cycles of proning.

His urine output declined, and he developed acute kidney injury. Overnight, his vasopressor requirements increased to 0.65 µg/kg/min of noradrenaline and 0.03 units/minute of vasopressin to maintain a mean arterial pressure (MAP) of >60 mmHg.

He was started on continuous veno-venous haemofiltration (CVVH) at 10:00 hrs.

The patient remained pyrexial with temperature readings of up to 41°C.

Serum potassium levels began to rise resulting in CVVH being adjusted to an enhanced rate.

You are called urgently to review the patient at 20:34 after he is found to be hypotensive with a blood pressure of 60/30 mmHg.

You perform an assessment of the patient, which is as follows:

Airway and breathing: Endotracheal tube *in-situ*, patient now in supine position, FIO_2 0.4, SpO_2 95%, PIP 24, PEEP 5, MV 9 L/min.

Circulation: Blood pressure 60/30 mmHg, heart rate 156 bpm. ECG (3-lead) reveals bizarre looking trace with broad QRS complexes.

Mottled skin with cool peripheries, central capillary refill time of 4 seconds.

Ongoing noradrenaline administration at a rate 1.2 µg/kg/min, and vasopressin at 0.04 units/minute.

Disability/CNS: On propofol 30 mg /hr (3.5 mg/kg/hr) alfentanil 4 ml/hr and rocuronium 5 ml/hr. Richmond agitation and sedation scale (RASS) = 4.

Blood glucose measured as 7.2 mmol/L.

Exposure: Nasogastric tube (NGT) *in-situ* with feed running. Last aspirate was recorded as being 250 ml.

Additional information—temperature 39.1°C.

Laboratory results from the morning as follows:

Urea and electrolytes; creatinine 500 µmol/L, urea 15 mg/dL, creatine kinase 500 U/L.

Full blood count—haemoglobin 117 g/L, white cell count 19 × 10^9/L, neutrophils 17 × 10^9/L

Urine output documented, 100 ml over the past 24 hours.

An arterial blood gas has been sent which reveals the following:

Time	17:00	19:13	Current (20:40)
pH	7.20	7.23	7.22
PaO_2	11	11.9	11.9
$PaCO_2$	5.5	5.0	4.8
Std Bicarb	15.4	15.8	14.8
BE	–11.5	–10.9	–12.3
Anion gap	22.8	21.3	26
FiO_2	.40	.4	.4
Na^-	134	134	130
K^+	5.6	6.3	8.3
Ca ions	0.95	0.85	0.86
Cl^-	101	103	99
Glucose	7.5	5.9	7.2
Lactate	1.1	1.54	3.9

What are the initial steps in the treatment of hyperkalaemia?

Ans: Hyperkalaemia ranges from mild to severe, with severe hyperkalaemia inferring a risk of life-threatening cardiac arrhythmias.[1] It is important to recognise myocardial excitability as a result of hyperkalaemia and treat it appropriately.

The patient described has severe hyperkalaemia (>6.5 mEq/L) with an unstable cardiac rhythm. Alongside treating the arrhythmia, emergency treatment for hyperkalaemia should be commenced.

The emergency management of severe hyperkalaemia with ECG changes is well outlined in the European Resuscitation Council (ERC) guidelines.[2]

This management approach consists of the administration of:

1. **Intravenous calcium:** Temporarily reduces myocardial excitability, therefore "protecting the heart". 10 ml of 10% calcium gluconate can be given over 5 minutes and repeated after 5 minutes if necessary (if there is evidence of persistent cardiac toxicity). 30 ml of 10% calcium chloride may also be used.
2. **Intravenous soluble insulin and glucose:** Reduces serum potassium concentration by shifting it intracellularly. 10 units of fast-acting insulin in 25 g glucose (e.g. 50 mL of 50% dextrose) given over 15–30 minutes.
3. **Nebulised salbutamol:** Reduces serum potassium by increasing cellular uptake of potassium. Effects last from around 30 minutes following administration, with a lower potassium level (by 0.5–1.0 mmol/L) maintained for up to a few hours. Administer 10–20 mg nebules through a breathing circuit.
4. **Potassium binders:** Sodium zirconium cyclosilicate and patiromer are selective potassium binders that do not result in the gastrointestinal effects associated with the use of older potassium binders. They remove excess potassium from the gastrointestinal tract. Their use is widely accepted in chronic hyperkalaemia but they are less-often used in acute hyperkalaemia. Serum potassium levels begin to decrease within 2 hours and normalise in 48 hours 95% of the time[3]. This is particularly useful in patients where electrolyte disturbances are likely to be prolonged.
5. **Renal replacement therapy (RRT):** The definitive method for removing excess potassium is by haemofiltration or dialysis.

What are the potential causes of hyperkalaemia in this patient?

Ans: The potential causes of hyperkalaemia are vast and it is often multifactorial.

In general, close consideration of the following aetiologies should be taken:

- **Renal causes**; AKI as a result of pre-renal failure, renal tubular acidosis, nephropathies, rhabdomyolysis and vasculitides. Renal failure was present in this case, but this itself would unlikely explain the current clinical picture without additional potassium administration or release as outlined below.
- **Drugs:** May impact potassium homeostasis via various mechanisms. These can be divided into:
  - Drugs which increase potassium efflux, including suxamethonium, beta-blockers, digoxin and mannitol. Also consider drugs causing apoptosis or cell destruction, such as propofol (as it is found in propofol infusion syndrome (PRIS)).
  - Drugs which reduce excretion, including mineralocorticoid receptor antagonists (such as spironolactone and eplerenone) and other potassium sparing diuretics.
  - Drugs that contain potassium, including incorrect administration of potassium supplements, low-sodium salt alternatives, and blood transfusions (via haemolysis).
- **Metabolic acidosis:** A low pH causes hydrogen ions to move intracellularly via hydrogen-potassium-ATPase ion pumps, resulting in an increase in plasma potassium levels.
- **Diabetic ketoacidosis (DKA) and hyperosmolar hyperglycaemic state (HHS):** As described above, hyperkalaemia occurs owing to the state of metabolic acidaemia. However, total potassium content is generally reduced, and falls quickly with treatment. Hypokalaemia is more often an issue with these patients owing to treatment with intravenous insulin infusion (which drives potassium into cells). Careful

potassium supplementation with close serum monitoring should be undertaken to ensure hyperkalaemia does not occur.

- **Rhabdomyolysis:** The breakdown of myocytes with subsequent potassium release into the plasma alongside the other intracellular components (mainly phosphate and uric acid). The mechanism of non-traumatic rhabdomyolysis is owing to ATP depletion in the myocyte which disables ion gradient mechanisms. The resulting accumulation of calcium in the sarcoplasm causes constant contraction, further ATP depletion, and destruction of the myocyte by activation of calcium-dependent neutral proteases and phospholipids.
- **Other, rarer considerations:** Adrenal disease (autoimmune, malignant), tumour lysis syndrome, pseudohyperkalaemia, uretojejunostomy, hyperkalaemic periodic paralysis).[1]

With reference to the case described, there is clear renal impairment (AKI) which could be a result of hypovolaemia in the context of sepsis, diarrhoea and fluid losses.

The medications listed do not directly alter potassium homeostasis, though there are two considerations. Propofol administration in the context of a raised creatine kinase (CK) could point toward PRIS. In reality, this patients sedation was changed to midazolam, and CK and triglycerides were re-checked.

The other consideration is the possibility of acute interstitial nephritis; a rare complication of the commonly used antibiotic piperacillin/tazobactam.[4]

This being said, the degree of hyperkalaemia is unlikely to be a result of renal failure alone, especially without potassium supplementation. As mentioned before, hyperkalaemia is often multifactorial[5] and a likely explanation is that the patient is in a state of rhabdomyolysis. Non-traumatic causes of rhabdomyolysis most commonly seen in intensive care include toxins, ischaemia, sepsis and hyperthermia,[6]of which the latter two are present in this patient.

It is important to note that AKI is present in up to 60% of rhabdomyolysis patients in the intensive care setting and can develop via several mechanisms.[7] This includes ischaemic tubular injury by way of myoglobin deposition in the renal microcirculation, reduced nitric oxide release and renin-angiotensin-aldosterone-system (RAAS) activation (alongside other vascular mediators) resulting in poor renal perfusion. Tubular obstruction from the formation of 'brown casts' (a result of acidic urine promoting interaction between myoglobin and Tamm-Horsfall proteins) also results in AKI and may be avoided by the administration of sodium bicarbonate to alkalinise the urine.

The diagnosis of rhabdomyolysis involves a CK of >5000 U/L. Myoglobin can be measured, but it is metabolized quickly and is therefore less reliable.

In this case the CK was repeated, revealing a rise to 85000 U/L, and despite aggressive initial management, plasma potassium remained high with haemodynamic instability and ECG changes for over 2 hours. Management of electrolyte disturbances in rhabdomyolysis is no mean feat; large volumes of fluid are required for adequate resuscitation owing to volume-depletion and sequestration by injured muscle. The aim is to produce large volumes of alkalinized urine (pH >6.5).

Unfortunately, in the presence of AKI with ongoing RRT, this was not achievable for this patient.

The mortality for a patient with rhabdomyolysis on intensive care is 22% without AKI, and as high as 59% with AKI.

2. CONTROVERSIAL ASPECTS OF MANAGEMENT "EVIDENCE CONTOUR"

Sodium bicarbonate is routinely recommended in cases of hyperkalemic cardiac arrest as described by the Resus Council UK. It acts by shifting potassium intracellularly, but it is not recommended in the routine treatment of hyperkalaemia. Studies are being conducted to assess if there is a role for it in the context of rhabdomyolysis and prevention of acute kidney injury.

Hyperventilation: This strategy may temporarily increase the pH, allowing potassium to shift intracellularily in exchange for hydrogen ions, however, excessive hyperventilation can result in reduced cerebral perfusion.

Running parallel filters/hd/changing dialysate fluid.

Calcium given in digitalis toxicity and the risk of 'stone heart': It was previously believed that calcium administration in the context of hyperkalaemia and digoxin toxicity could result in cardiac arrest. This has not been shown in studies and, in a retrospective study by Levine et al, concluded that calcium should not be delayed due to fear of this phenomenon. (Levine et al. 2011)

Mannitol in rhabdomyolysis—if there remains a low urine output

PRIS—regular monitoring and alternatives

DIABETIC KETOACIDOSIS

A 19-year-old woman presents to the emergency department after 4 days of nausea and vomiting. She has diarrhoea and is complaining of intense thirst. She is unsure if she has taken her insulin.

Her mother brings her in as she has become drowsy and her home glucose monitoring is reading 'high'.

Her initial venous blood gas shows a pH of 7.02, $PaCO_2$ 3.2, HCO_3 of 5 and ketones of 6.7, potassium of 3.

What are the indications of severe DKA? Which cases would require high dependency treatment?

Features which represent severe DKA and possible need for critical care support include:[8]

- Oxygen saturations <92%
- Tachycardia or bradycardia
- Systolic blood pressure <90 mmHg after initial fluid resuscitation
- Serum potassium <3.5 mmol/L on admission
- Urine output <0.5 ml/kg/hr
- Blood ketones >6.0 mmol/L
- Venous pH <7.0
- Venous bicarbonate <5 mmol/L
- Anion gap >16
- GCS less than 12
- High risk patient groups, e.g. those who are pregnant or suffer with renal failure or heart failure.

Evidence Contour

1. *Rate of Fixed Insulin Infusion*

The standard practice advises that the rate of insulin infusion starts at 0.1 unit/kg/hour. There is a significant incidence of hypokalaemia and hypoglyceamia seen in this population—mainly caused by insulin administration.

An RCT performed in children demonstrated no significant increase in time to resolution of DKA with 0.05 units/kg/hr in comparison to 0.1 unit/kg/hour, however, the risk of hypoglycaemia was reduced from 20% to 4% and hypokalaemia was reduced from 48% to 20% with lower insulin infusion rates. This has been replicated in our studies.

The JBDS-IP has now recommended that the rate of insulin infusion should be commenced at 0.1 unit/kg/hour, but should drop to 0.05 units/kg/hour once blood sugar drops to <14 mmol/L9.

2. *Normal Saline vs Balanced Crystalloid*

Balanced crystalloid such as Hartmann's solution may not be as common on general medical wards and contains potassium, but not in sufficient concentration for most DKA patients and does not come pre-mixed. The UK NPSA recommends that solutions containing potassium are premixed to avoid dosing errors which can lead to death. Saline bags are available with pre-mixed potassium in various concentrations.

Hartmann's solution is also thought to risk worsening acidosis through its bicarbonate, increase the already raised lactate pyruvate ratio in DKA and potentially worsen cerebral oedema as it is hypotonic.[10] In comparison, 0.9% sodium chloride contains more chloride and can result in renal vasoconstriction and oliguria due to hyperchloraemic metabolic acidosis. This can prolong recovery from DKA.[9]

There have been two randomised controlled trials which showed no difference in clinical outcomes initially, however, in post-hoc analysis, faster resolution of DKA was found with balanced crystalloid, but only in a critical care environment.[8]

The most recent systematic review (Jan 22) revealed longer time to resolution of DKA and longer hospital stays with normal saline in comparison to balanced crystalloid.

3. *IV Bicarbonate*

According to recent guidelines from JBDS-IP 2021, intravenous bicarbonate is not recommended as in the systematic review showed only improvement of metabolic acidosis in the first two hours, but difference to glycaemic control or clinical improvement. However, in the case of concurrent disease or pH <6.85, it may be considered.

In the paediatric population, IV bicarbonate has been linked to higher rates of cerebral oedema and increased length of stay in retrospective studies.

No adult studies reported cerebral oedema.[8]

4. *Venous vs arterial blood gas sampling*

Pain for the patient is reduced, and in the context of multiple admissions for many patients, repeated arterial blood sampling may result in delayed presentation to secondary care. Risks of complications like vascular occlusion are reduced.

Studies comparing pH and bicarbonate results in patients presenting with DKA and without have shown that there is very little difference.[11] For $PaCO_2$, there was more variance, however, a value of <6 kPa rules out clinically significant hypercapnoea with 100% sensitivity in a study looking at 529 patients. Base excess varied with inconsistent results, however, lactate shows a general agreement when comparing normal *vs* raised lactate.[8]

Venous blood gas is widely used for patients in DKA, however, if the results do not correlate with the clinical picture, or if there are increasing oxygen requirements, an arterial blood gas should be performed.[11]

5. *Community Treatment for Mild DKA*

Although in the UK, patients with any degree of DKA are treated in a hospital setting, protocols exist in other countries to include the use of oral fluids and subcutaneous rapid acting insulin within pre-defined biochemical parameters.[12]

6. *Phosphate Replacement*

Phosphate is normally depleted in the setting of DKA, even when initial serum tests are unremarkable. This could lead to respiratory failure, rhabdomyolysis and cardiac arrhythmia and should be supplemented in cases of severe hypophosphatemia where this is a risk. However, there is no evidence to recommend routine replacement of phosphate in DKA.[2]

Final points

1. Hyperkalemia is life threatening and should be managed immediately without delay.
2. A protocolized management always improves outcome.
3. Bicarbonate is a double edged sword and has to be used with caution.
4. Hypophosphatemia is not so uncommon in DKA and is one of the causes of weaning failure.
5. Balance salt solution may be an effective alternative to normal saline in fluid replacement during DKA management.

REFERENCES

1. Yarlagadda S, Assessment of hyperkalaemia. BMJ Best Practice. Bestpractice.bmj.com accessed 08 October 2022, last updates 25 Feb 2022.
2. Lott C, Truhlář A, Alfonzo A, et al. European Resuscitation Council Guidelines 2021: Cardiac arrest in special circumstances. Resuscitation. 2021 Apr;161:152–219. Full text (https://www.doi.org/10.1016/j.resuscitation.2021.02.011)
3. Deakin c, Soar J, Davies R. Resuscitation Council UK. Special circumstances guidelines. May 2021[internet publication]. Full text https://www.resus.org.uk/library/2021-resuscitation-guidelines/specialcircumstancesguidelines)
4. Richard R Watkins, Stan Deresinski, Increasing Evidence of the Nephrotoxicity of Piperacillin/Tazobactam and Vancomycin Combination Therapy—What Is the Clinician to Do?, Clinical Infectious Diseases, Volume 65, Issue 12, 15 December 2017, Pages 2137–2143, https://doi.org/10.1093/cid/cix675)
5. Abuelo JG. Treatment of Severe Hyperkalemia: Confronting 4 Fallacies. Kidney Int Rep. 2017 Oct 7;3(1):47–55. doi: 10.1016/j.ekir.2017.10.001. PMID: 29340313; PMCID: PMC5762976
6. Torres PA, Helmstetter JA, Kaye AM, Kaye AD. Rhabdomyolysis: pathogenesis, diagnosis, and treatment. Ochsner J. 2015 Spring;15(1):58-69. PMID: 25829882; PMCID: PMC436584
7. Saxena P, Dhooria S, Agarwal R, Prasad KT, Sehgal IS. Rhabdomyolysis in Intensive Care Unit: More than One Cause. Indian J Crit Care Med. 2019 Sep;23(9):427-429. doi: 10.5005/jp-journals-10071-23238. PMID: 31645829; PMCID: PMC6775710.
8. Rayman G, Diabetic Ketoacidosis. BMJ Best Practice. Bestpractice.bmj.com BMJ Publishing Group Ltd 2022. accessed 08 October 2022, last update 19 July 2022.

9. Joint British Diabetes Societies for Inpatient Care(JBDS-IP). The management of diabetic ketoacidosis in adults. June 2021 [internet publication].
10. Dhatariya KK. Diabetic ketoacidosis. BMJ. 2007 Jun 23;334(7607):1284-5. Abstract.
11. Kelly AM. Can VBG analysis replace ABG analysis in emergency care? Emerg Med J. 2016 Feb;33(2):152–4. Abstract.
12. Karslioglu French E, Donihi AC, Korytkowski MT. Diabetic ketoacidosis and hyperosmolar hyperglycemic syndrome: review of acute decompensated diabetes in adult patients. BMJ. 2019 May 29;365:l1114. Full text Abstract.

CHAPTER

21

The Diagnosis Process in Intensive Care Unit

Jorge Hidalgo, Allyson Hidalgo

ABSTRACT

Most patients admitted to the medical Intensive Care Units (ICUs) have common diseases. As physicians, our training is to identify a single explanation for our patient's medical condition; the more accurate our diagnosis is, the more effective the medical management.

However, a group of patients presents with a challenging clinical scenario. However, they have some physiological alterations that require the response of the ICU team and give supportive management, such as fluids due to hypotension and proper monitoring due to alterations in the mental status and hemodynamic instability, among other things. This patient needs help establishing the etiology since there is no significant information. Generally, they will get admitted to the ICU and can go their entire admission course without a diagnosis.

Patient with difficult diagnosis increase the morbidity and mortality and represent a challenge for the team. If a diagnosis is made, a proper plan and course of management and treatment can be done. The patients that recover without a diagnosis give us a sense that the work is incomplete.

The truth is that every day we face a very complex medical case. Whether it is because modern patients are more complicated or because in the setting of critical illness, diagnosis is more complex, or because we all claimed to be busy. We are not spending time taking a medical history and conducting a proper physical exam.

▪ ***Keywords:*** *Difficult cases, Physical Exam, Team Approach, Proper communication, Unknown.*

CLINICAL SCENARIO

A 45-year-old male patient, African-American descendent, who lives in Belmopan City, a primary school teacher, who initially visits the emergency room for a generalized malaise and fatigue, complaining of a 7-day history of fever. PMH: medical history is unremarkable, he is a social drinker, nonsmoker. Covid-19 fully vaccinated. Present physical exam: VS: BP: 100/60 HR:110 RR:20 SPO_2: 99 RA, he is alert, not in respiratory distress, and has moderate dehydration. He got a mild COVID without the need for hospitalization.

Neck: Supple, no lymphadenopathy. RT-PCR-Covid-19 are negative. Weight 72.3 kg. and Height: 5'9"

Heart: RRR, Normal S1/S2, No S3S4, No R/G/M Normal Peripheral Pulses, No pedal edema

Chest: Clear breath sounds bilaterally

Abdomen: Soft, nondistended, (+) BS, no rebound.

Neuro: No focal. The patient starts on resuscitation fluids, blood cultures are taken, and he is started with broad-spectrum antibiotics, lactate: 5. Initial WBC, BUN/Creatinine, and comprehensive liver function are negative. Malaria, Dengue, Zika, Chikungunya, and widal are negative. Chest X-ray normal, and EKG except for sinus tachycardia; the rest is normal. The patient continues to deteriorate rapidly and is transferred to the general ICU for proper hemodynamic monitoring. After 48 hours, the patient still with a persistent fever. His vital signs are more stable; however, he is still on a low-dosage drip of norepinephrine. The initial urinary, stool and blood cultures report negatives. In addition, a contrasted CT scan of the thorax/abdomen/pelvis was reported normal. The medical history was reviewed. We emphasized travel history, special adventure tours visiting caves, the presence of pigeons or other pets at home, and exposure to ticks. He denies exposure to other animals except his dog (fully immunized). After seven days in ICU, the patient management is supportive, and we cannot conclude any diagnosis. The only new development is two episodes of supraventricular tachycardia. Electrolytes are normal. The case was brought to discussion with the medical department to decide the next step on the approach to this challenging case.

Key Point: A proper careful medical history and complete physical exam must be performed, with questions related to past medical—surgical and nonsurgical procedures. Another question that is also important is the presence or not of foreign bodies or implants, any condition that leads to immunosuppression, and travel history—the exposure to animals and if there are any diet habits and list of medication.

Clinical decision-making and applying the reasoning process to a patient clinical scenario are essential skills in clinical practice. There are two ways we usually use in the decision-making process:

a. Dual-Process theory: This is an intuitive, pattern-based approach—a better example is the instant recognition of a skin rash like chickenpox.
b. Analytical, rule-based approach. This is more complex, including hypothetic-deductive reasoning.

Many of our clinical decisions utilize both systems, and it is challenging to establish the system the clinician uses.[1]

The ICU patient: In ICU, our immediate approach is to focus on the physiological changes that can comprise our patient's life. Once the patient is stable, we must work to establish the diagnosis; however, we are constantly working on the most common medical problems. So to approach the uncommon diagnosis, the workflow that we usually use needs to change, and we need to back to the patient over and over, taking a detailed medical history and doing a complete physical exam as often as needed.

How we can identified the challenge cases, it is impossible. The most logical approach is to rule out the most frequent medical diagnosis, and after that, we can think of those that are less common. Once we complete this exercise and have not seen any improvement in our patients, we need to do the differential diagnosis exercise based on the epidemiological information.[1,2]

Key Point: When caring for patients in general, we need to offer the highest value in a personalized manner that delivers proven benefits and minimizes the risk and unnecessary associated expenses.

We need to place our patients' care, outcomes, values, and concerns at the center of every major clinical decision and involve the patients and families in the process. Based on Evidence-based medical information.

In the beginning, it is challenging to establish whether the patient is presenting with an uncommon diagnosis. We must stress to the team that in those cases, we need to review the medical history and the physical exam looking for signs and symptoms that lead us to the diagnosis (elimination approach). Inaccurate working diagnosis, most of the time, could be harmful. It is essential to go back many times as needed and try to see the patient with a fresh eye.

In this model approach, an essential component is obtaining information on recent admission and also from the primary care clinic; of course, this process is time-consuming and rewarding.

Having a diagnosis is critical to make the plan of management and treatment and will help us reduce admission time, morbidity, and mortality. If we need a diagnostic test that will be confirmed or rule out a possible diagnosis, we must get it done. This is a team effort and multidisciplinary approach, most of the time calling for those specialties from which the patient will benefit. We need to understand that those complex cases imply cycles of hypothesis, sometimes with uncertainty accumulating room for error.

In this case, it can become frustrating for the team and surrounded by a lack of objectivity.[1,2]

In this circumstance, the personalities, the proactivity, and the team taking care of the patient are critical; we need to have a high index of suspicion. We need to seek new information and clues that allow us to generate hypotheses to look for. Consultants are most valuable in investigating and confirming diagnosis once it has been proposed.[2,3]

Clinical Aspects to have in Consideration in the ICU Setting

The clinicians are challenged to understand the significance of the signs and symptoms and the role of the test in the clinical approach. We must remember that unnecessary tests increase the cost, and we must utilize those strategies with the best diagnostic value.[2,3]

Key Point: A thorough medical history taken along generates the highest diagnostic information along with a physical exam.

The medical condition affecting the patient must be capable of causing critical illness or tend to coexist with diseases that do. Clinicians must address the symptoms in a focused manner and review the previous diagnosis diligently. The findings should guide the additional testing and should use consultation with other specialties judiciously.

The ICU population varies, from those that have simple medical condition, to those that have an important medical background: Chronic kidney disease, diabetes, heart problems among other, and most of the time are with a extensive list of medication.[2,3,4]

A. Most frequent medical condition
B. And the question: Are we facing a challenge diagnosis?
C. We must start from the beginning, revisiting the differential diagnosis based on the new information and continuously collecting data.

It is important to go through the information obtained during this admission and any other data from a recent one, including previous testing, exposure, therapeutical trials, and any clue that can help with the diagnosis.[2,3,4]

The main goal of a patient admitted into the ICU with a difficult diagnosis is restoring function and integrating the patient into his social life.

Table 21.1: List of difficult medical problems by system

Neurological diseases	***Cardiovascular diseases***
These usually cause encephalopathy, odd focal deficits, or neuromuscular weakness.	These tend to be a cause of refractory shock
Psychogenic signs and symptoms, acute disseminated encephalomyelitis, acute cerebellar ataxia, optic neuromyelitis, transverse myelitis, demyelinating neuropathy, cytomegalovirus-related radiculitis, Lyme disease, metabolic and electrolyte disorders, porphyria, botulism, myasthenia gravis, acute inflammatory myopathies, mitochondrial myopathies, Guillain-Barré	Sepsis and systemic inflammatory response syndrome, spinal cord trauma, anaphylaxis, toxic shock syndrome, adrenal crisis, mixedematous coma, myocardial infarction, idiopathic myocardiopathy, blunt cardiac trauma, constrictive pericarditis.
The difficult weaning	***Gastrointestinal diseases***
Weaning from ventilator challenges.	The difficult diagnosis
In most of the patients, we must use weaning predictors to identify those potential patients suitable for weaning or to confirm lack of readiness to wean.	Celiac disease, pancreatic exocrine insufficiency, inflammatory bowel disease, intermittent porphyria
Kidney diseases	***Hematology and oncology***
Renal failure difficult diagnosis	There are variety of hematology disorders that represent a challenge
Obstructive nephropathy Acute interstitial nephritis	The oncology immunosuppressed patient with an atypical presentation.
Autoimmunne related nephropathies	Platelet-related disorders
	Transplant patient
Endoncrine	***Infectious diseases***
The atypical presentation of acute complication of DM II.	Unknown origin fever
Thyroid related condition	Marburg, Ebola fever
Pancreatic disorders	Atypical presentation of bacteria, viral, fungal infection
Drug overdose and toxicology	***Other conditions***
Very common in our days	
Design drugs (specially in patients coming from night clubs)	Newly emerging infectious disease
Opioids (Fentanyl abuse)	
Lead poisoning	

The Values

A. We need to show a profound respect for our patient.
B. Competence and compassion.
C. The ability to conduct a proper history taking and do a good physical examination are Important in the diagnosis process. The history and physical exam are inseparable.
D. Technology cannot replace the physician; it is what you do that builds a trusting, fruitful relationship with the patient.[5]

This framework is evolving. Have a high index of suspicion is critical in the diagnosis process. As clinicians, we know how to take a good medical history and complement it with a thorough physical exam supplemented by guided additional laboratories, imaging among others to guide the treatment and management possibilities.

REFERENCES

1. K. Sundsted. D. Bierle, et al. Clinical Decision Making and Interpreting the Medical literature. MKSAP19. American College of Physician 2021.
2. Brandon Otto. Difficult Diagnoses in the ICU. Critical Concepts, meditations on critical illness. http://critcon.org/archives/1086. April 19, 2021.
3. K.L Singer. Difficult Medical Management. New England Journal of Medicine. 1991; 324:1601–1601.
4. A.L. Komaroff, T.F. Landsdale III. Difficult Diagnosis 2. New England Journal of Medicine, 1993; 328:68–69.
5. H. Seidel, J Ball, J Dains. The history and interviewing process. Mosby guide to Physical Examination. Mosby Elsevier 2006. PP 2–37.

Index